Hormone Basics

Every woman's guide to health and happiness for the body, mind, and spirit

I've had the pleasure of being a colleague of Dr. Leatherman's for several years and congratulate him on the user-friendly and highly instructional nature of Hormone Basics. *This book is needed.*

In addition to being a true healer through chiropractic and acupuncture, Dr. Leatherman has done an incredible job with his first book for the purpose of educating and informing. Hormone Basics *is thorough, but light, an approach that makes it easy to learn about the importance of hormones for the maintenance of good health. Dr. Leatherman provides a unique outlook on the current state of hormonal imbalance in the general population and how the facts on this topic generally remain hidden and go uncorrected in our modern yet traditional medical offices and homes. This perspective is key to understanding how we can all change our lives for the better; integral to this understanding is knowing what constitutes a healthy diet, how to avoid a toxic lifestyle, and the facts of general nutrition…all topics included in this comprehensive guide.*

I am pleased to be a friend of Dr. Chris Leatherman and hope to join him in spreading his message of health and healing to all those in need.

Bravo, Dr. Chris, keep up your great works!

– Edward W. Pearson, M.D., ABIHM, Founder
New Medicine Foundation, 2010

Hormone Basics *is full of great, timely information. I don't think the public can get enough of it to help them make better decisions about their hormones and health.*

– Eric Everett, R.Ph., Certified Clinical Nutritionist, 2010

Hormone Basics

Every woman's and girl's guide

to health and happiness for the

body, mind, and spirit

Dr. Chris Leatherman

Published by Princeton-Hudson Communications, LLC

Kansas City, MO

Printed in the United States of America

ISBN13: 978-0-9826792-0-3

Library of Congress Control Number: 2010942954

Book orders: please go to www.hormonebasics.com

Editing, cover artwork, and book design by

Harvard Girl Word Services · www.harvardgirledits.com

Dedication

This book is for my mother. Keep your faith, Mom. Keep doing your best to stay positive for all of us the way you always have. I hope today is a good day and wish you a lifetime of good days.

This book is also for my wife Kylee with whom I celebrated our seventh wedding anniversary last December. Our best year yet, they keep getting better, especially since the birth of our son Robert Christopher last April. For me to try to explain how I feel for Kylee would diminish the feeling, so I won't try. I have never met a woman so loving, beautiful, passionate, strong, intelligent, funny, caring, and thoughtful. And that's just the beginning. Kylee, thank you for being my best friend, for caring for me, supporting me, and giving me guidance when you know I need it—and especially when I don't realize I do. Thank you for accepting my faults and loving me more for them. I am truly blessed to have you in my life; I am a better man for it.

And finally, this book is for my daughter. Alex, what can I say? I've always tried to do my best for you, even when I couldn't be there as much as we wanted. How you live from your soul and continue to grow through your heart will always inspire me. You have a gift; continue to follow it. You will always have the best of my love and spirit.

Acknowledgments

Thanks to my sister Keri who has inspired me in my passion to help people. I wish for you only healthy, pain-free days. I see you in so many of my patients and that makes me want to help them even more. I don't tell you often enough that I love you.

As much as we might love our parents, spouse, or another person, we only learn about true, unconditional love when we have a child. This kind of love is a love from the soul, from the original source; it knows no limits and starts before the child is born. I believe this love never dies, even when we do. This is the love I have for my daughter Alex and son Bobby; I wish them both lifetimes of health and happiness.

I also want to express my gratitude to the colleagues and friends who helped me during a very difficult time in my life. These friends provided more than a place to sleep and study; they saved me from going off the deep end when I felt totally lost and on a couple of occasions likely saved my life. Without them I could not have succeeded. So, thanks again, Joel, Pat, Courtenay, Erica, Mike, Jeremy, and Adrien.

Table of Contents

Introduction

How Being Ignored Can Kill You

If there is one single message in this book it is this: when you live the life you were gifted to live, you will love the life you are living. But the sad truth is that if you are one of the approximately 54 million women in this country who are between the ages of 14 and 44, you may *not* love the life you are living. In fact, you may not feel you are really "living" at all.

It may be hard to imagine that 54 million women between the ages of 14 and 44 have something significant in common. We all know it's not race or religion—and it certainly isn't a similar taste in fashion. But the answer is something that might surprise you because the unfortunate truth is this: If you are a female in this age group, you, and the other 53,999,999 women with you, are being unequivocally and fundamentally overlooked by the health care system. That's right: in terms of your health, *you are being ignored.*

You probably want to know what leads me to make such a strong statement. First of all, as a medical practitioner I know a lot about our current health care system. I know that unless you are in the group of women who are approximately 44 and over and going through "the change" (menopause) or consciously trying to "balance your hormones," it's likely that you'll have to wait until you reach that phase of your life before you will have any real contact with this not-so-caring health care system.

That's why most women will not have access to the kind of care they need until they are well into their 40s. Millions of you, girls and women after the age of about 14 and through the age of the onset of menopause, are being left completely to your own devices by a health care system governed by tunnel vision. It is my opinion that such an oversight keeps you waiting much too long to be recognized, especially if you're just hitting puberty now and menopause is light years away. Waiting for such a long time without access to the right kind of information, and weighed down by the responsibility of having to figure things out alone, can make you feel lost. Precisely when you need the appropriate resources to understand yourself, your body, and what you feel, the health care system as we know it is leaving you out in the cold.

I wrote this book so you can come in from the cold. To allow you to stop feeling you have to sort out everything solo. To provide options to help you see things differently. To offer suggestions that may help you start to love your life—or love your life a whole lot more. Because I think the moment you start to really love your life is the moment you will truly begin to live.

From strife to life

When life doesn't feel like a "gift" it can feel like a struggle. Struggling through life often leads to a sense of disappointment and being perpetually disappointed can spawn the expectation that life delivers more suffering than enjoyment. Habitual sadness, loneliness, pain, or depression can make life feel a lot more like a burden than a joy. And honestly, if life feels oppressive for long enough it can feel more like a slow death than a life. Believe it or not, many women actually feel this way for days, months, years—even decades—and the vast majority accept their circumstances simply because they don't know how to change them.

As I said, there *is* something that shifts this trend, but unfortunately it doesn't usually happen until a woman hits her 40s. Why do things change so radically with the approach of menopause? Because in a sort of miraculous turn-around, the millions of women who have been so egregiously ignored by the health care system for most of their lives suddenly find themselves appearing as bright blips on the system's radar screen. This shift in attention has a significant and profound effect because after years of wearing virtual cloaks of invisibility these women finally begin to achieve visibility status in the eyes of the system. At long last they are presented with the chance to get the attention and care they need.

How should you feel about this gross negligence? I'd say outraged. Because whether you are 14 or 114, you are neither too young or too old to learn what you need to know to live a healthy life. You should not have to wait for a day or a month, let alone 40 or more years!

That's where the information in this book enters the picture. The more you understand the ideas presented here, the better you will be able to protect yourself from the things that may be contributing to how you feel about your body and your life. These things include hormonal imbalances, the environmental factors that contribute to their production, and many of the numerous dangerous side effects these imbalances can produce. I would ask you to bear in mind as you read that this information is not only for you, but for all the women you love and care about: your daughters, sisters, nieces, aunts, mothers, grandmothers, and friends. If you do happen to be the mother of a daughter, there is never a better time than the present to educate yourself about hormones in preparation for educating her.

It has become very apparent to me over the years, especially as my daughter Alex has matured, that horrible oversights have been occurring for generations…probably for centuries. When I ask women what they know about hormones their typical response is, "Not much. What I know I got in a video in junior high." Some of these women's moms advised them that they would be going through a "change," that is, that their menstrual cycle would begin, but these were the fortunate ones. Typically, women have been prone to share very little about their own experience of getting their periods for the first time and even less about the physical and emotional symptoms that naturally occur as part of the process.

Please know that it is not my goal to place blame! Every mom, aunt, sister, and grandmother does her absolute best to handle what might be an uncomfortable topic. But even if she doesn't shy away from detailed conversations about menstruation, puberty, and sex, the topic of hormones undoubtedly goes unmentioned. Why? I believe it's simply because you can't teach what you don't know.

Why hormones matter

Frankly, I'm not so sure that the subject of hormones shouldn't be a required course in our schools, if only to give all women a fighting chance to know what they are up against. But since my dream of educating the masses may never come true, I'm going to start here with the facts about hormones and what makes them so important.

Without getting too technical, hormones are tiny chemical powerhouses of information and energy. These powerhouses are vital, interactive "links" between our cells and every other part of our body. These links ultimately determine how well our body works (how healthy we are) or how poorly our body works (how unwell we are), depending on how well they are doing their job. Hormones are doubly important because they contribute to every aspect of bodily function and, therefore, to every aspect of life as we know it. It is interesting, therefore, that although hormones affect us in big ways and small ways, and although their effects are constant, we tend not to concern ourselves with them—as long as they keep doing what they are supposed to do. This is not unusual behavior. Most of us expect our bodies to serve our needs. It is only when the message we get is other than what we want to hear that we are forced to pay closer attention. In effect, we ignore the things that may not be "quite right" until we just can't ignore them anymore.

It's a bit like going to the dentist with a cavity. Most of us know that when we feel pain there is a problem and that it is time to make a call. Unfortunately, hormones don't always "tell us" when something is wrong so clearly. Symptoms of a hormonal imbalance may come and go, lessen and increase in severity, or even disappear altogether for a periods of time. This can cause us to not trust what we feel. But if we do not choose to listen to what our hormones are trying to tell us over a long enough time, eventually we will be forced to listen.

Chances are you fall into one of two categories. Either you have never paid much attention to hormones and have no idea why you should start now, or you are somewhere on the scale of discontented to miserable and you're wondering what's going on, but you don't know what to do about it.

Either way, whether you believe it or not, what you don't know about your hormones can hurt you. Hormones that aren't functioning correctly can make you unhappy or sick. They can even kill you if the malfunctioning goes on long enough. (Trust me; I know.) That's why the first step to changing anything is education. In this case, a lack of education about your hormones and their powerful link to your health gives them power they shouldn't have to control you and every aspect of your life. And I am a firm believer that YOU should be the one in control, not the other way around.

The great news is that once you learn certain facts about your health and hormones and start making choices based on your knowledge, you will start to feel amazing. And when you feel great you will also feel empowered to live a longer, healthier, and happier life.

This book has been written to provide answers to questions you may not even know you have. It will provide you with a better understanding of what your hormones are all about, preferably before they create what might seem like a lifetime of unanswerable questions and complications. This book has also been written as a vehicle for my message to every woman out there: that there *is* hope, that it *is* possible for you to feel good, and that feeling good can come from understanding more about your hormones.

What this does *not* mean is that the next 200-plus pages are full of hard-to-understand scientific information. For as complicated as hormones are in a biological sense, their roles and effects are pretty easy to understand. And it is my belief that once you understand the basics about your hormones, you will be able to start living the life you were gifted to live—and love every minute of it.

PART ONE

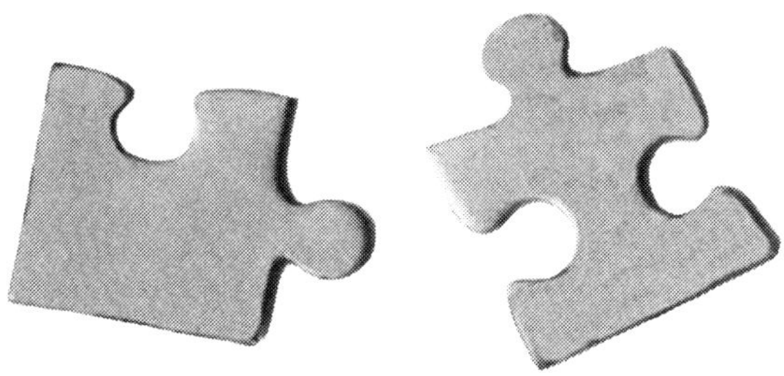

Hormone Basics

1

What's Missing & Why I Did It

If you have spent as much time looking for books about hormones as I have, you've been disappointed. Sure, you've probably found plenty of books on menopause (the cessation of the menstrual cycle), and admittedly these are extremely helpful for those suffering from the sometimes debilitating effects from the hormonal imbalances that go along with it. You've probably also found a number of books aimed at girls going through their "first change," or puberty, and the onset of menstruation. And if one wants to get lost in scientific jargon and biology lessons, books abound on the subject of the female anatomy. Granted, in many cases, these books are valuable sources of information that provide guidance and insight, but where are the books for everyone in between? Where is the down-to-earth information we need for the rest of the female population: those who don't fit neatly into one extreme stage (puberty) or the other (menopause)? Where are the guidelines for the approximately 54 million women between the ages of 14 and 44—like you?

I'll tell you. Nowhere.

It turns out that the reason you and I haven't been able to locate books that focus on this particular subject is because they are virtually nonexistent. Books that bridge the gap of information relative to this specific time frame for women and that can be used as easy-access reference guides simply cannot be found. That's why I decided I needed to write one myself. At the very least, I believe that no matter what age you are, you deserve to know everything you need to know about something that is so vital to every aspect of your body's ability to function and on every aspect of your daily life. What is that something? Hormones.

As females, hormones are active participants in your happiest and most joyous occasions. They may also be the underlying cause for some of the worst, possibly even life threatening, events you may experience in your lifetime. My goal, in attempting to keep potentially complicated, confusing, and complex information simple, basic, and accurate, is to provide a springboard for you to begin to have the confidence to ask more questions of yourselves and your health care providers.

I believe this information on hormones is so basic that even a guy can understand it. Well...maybe not. Because as confusing and frustrating as hormones are for girls and women, they are an even bigger mystery to us guys. To be honest, I felt that if I could write a book about hormones that made sense to guys, it would be a cakewalk for those of the female persuasion.

Just so you know, too, one of the driving forces behind the writing of this book is the special connection I have always had with women. This connection goes much deeper than the typical boy/girl connection that starts back in elementary school. You know the one, where the girls chase the boys and get to kiss them when they catch them. Well, it didn't take long for me to figure out the benefits of this game and let's just say that I prided myself at being the slowest boy on the playground. If the game were an Olympic event I'd have been a gold medalist. With that said, the connection I feel is much more meaningful than having, needing, or wanting a girlfriend or wife. It's difficult, but I'll do my best to explain.

I have always sensed that women emit a different kind of energy and for some reason I seem to be able to pick up on this energy and respond to it in a way that is automatic, straight from the heart, and honest. Please understand that this has absolutely nothing to do with anything physical whatsoever. It simply means that as long as I've been alive I have been comfortable in the midst of the female gender. In fact, my wife Kylee is the first to admit I typically fit just as easily into a gathering of "the girls" as I do one with the guys.

Whether it's out in public among women I've never met, in the clinic with patients, or among friends, my heightened sensitivity to both the beauty and the pain experienced by the women in my life is apparent. No, I'm not a mind reader and no, it's not like *What Women Want,* the movie where Mel Gibson can hear what women are thinking. This is more about a feeling I get from women, as if they're sending out signals about whether they're happy—or not; whether they're feeling good—or are in pain. Unfortunately, I often get the distinct impression that they are not only in pain, but sad as well, with a liberal dose of frustration and limitation to boot. And it's all topped with a shroud of what many of them have described to me as a "living in a fog." I personally believe that many times these girls and women know there is something missing from their lives, that there is something more to who and what they are, but they can't figure out who or what that is. I also feel that no matter how they might see themselves or explain themselves, when it comes to women I have been given the gift of insight. I see them for how wonderful they really are, both inside and out. Why? I don't have a clue.

For years I secretly watched *Oprah* and other shows that focused on women and women's issues. For a long time, *Oprah* was the only show host who consistently delved into women's deepest needs and desires, so it was from her show that I got a lot of my early clues. I also admit to being the unlikely guy in the waiting room reading *Self* instead of *Popular Mechanics*, scouring the pages for insight into how and what women thought (though I occasionally resorted to camouflage, hiding *O* or *Women's Day* inside a hunting or car magazine). But I needed to learn more about what really interested me:

women. Who they were, what they were, how they thought and felt, and why.

More about me

A little background about me might be helpful here. I grew up your typical all-American farm boy. I spent many of my days on a tractor hauling hay, building fences, hunting, fishing, and playing sports. When the time came, I was the Prince of the Prom, too. I tried hard to adhere to the stereotypical role of a macho guy's guy and for the most part managed pretty well. But to be honest, it felt pretty limiting given how conscious I was of my empathy for the other half of the human race. Naturally, I was uncomfortable expressing this "compassionate interest" too openly for many years. But I didn't let it stop me from discovering as much as I could about the dramatic and intriguing differences between women and men. In fact, I became more intent on finding the answers I sought as time went on.

In great part it was my mother who was the seed for the journey I have traveled. I don't remember a time when she wasn't plagued from the ravages of health issues, many of which, it turns out, were hormonal. It would be years before I would begin to understand the complex circumstances that led to her difficulties. Today, though much improved, my mother continues to experience such health "problems." But the afflictions she faced on a daily basis for so long pained me as her child, and the pain of a child unable to help his mother has never left me. As a kid all I wanted was for my mom to feel good. I didn't understand what was wrong and certainly had no idea what to do about it. But I thought that maybe if she felt good for one day she could feel good for two; if she felt good for two days then maybe she could feel good for an entire week or an entire month. I wish I could say that was how it went. But it didn't. And after years of questioning why and getting no real answers in return, my frustration peaked. So, at least to some degree, this book is the result of my search for an explanation.

What I knew then on a subconscious level and know now as a grown man is that we all deserve what my mother deserves: to know what it is like to live without pain, without the sense that something is "wrong" with her. She deserves to be able to wake up in the morning and not dread the day because she is already worn out, has a headache, has a stomach ache or an intestinal "issue," or any number of other problems. She shouldn't have to decide how to organize her day based on whether she is having a flare-up of her chronic fatigue or fibromyalgia or any of the other conditions that continue to afflict her to some degree even now. She should be able to be herself and to enjoy the things she has fun doing. Instead, Mom has spent the majority of her life trying to figure out what was wrong with her and why she always felt so bad.

My mother's health, or lack thereof, has been a source of confusion, mystery, and distress. Obviously, writing this book may not cure my mother's or anyone else's difficulties. But maybe if she'd had a better understanding when she was younger about certain aspects of her health (in this case about her hormones and stress), hers might have been an easier path.

I see everyday how women—and the people who love them—suffer with the same challenges…and it is not okay with me.

Furthermore, as the brother of a sister who shares many of our mother's health challenges, I have yet another reason to do what I can to make things better. I have the utmost love, respect, admiration, and pride for my sister Keri as the mother of two and a successful businesswoman—especially in light of the way she faces her challenges with the same courage, tolerance, and patience as our mother always did—but I have always wanted to do more to help.

As a husband and father, I also feel a deep responsibility to my daughter Alex and my wife Kylee. I know I am already late putting this information in book form for Alex, who just turned fifteen, but hopefully it's never too late. Even though Alex has already begun to experience many of the changes all girls experience, if she can grasp just a portion of what's in this book and hold on to it, perhaps her life (and the lives of other girls like her) will be a little better.

As for my wife, I have never met a woman who is more dedicated to her overall health. Kylee watches with care everything she puts in or on her body. Her dedication to living a healthy lifestyle, which includes the practice of yoga, is nothing short of amazing. Kylee is like many women who have had their fair share of challenges with health and hormones, but she has never given up. She never accepted "I don't know" or "It's all in your head" as an answer, though there were times that would have been the easiest thing to do. Instead, she has never left a stone unturned in her quest for the best health she can achieve and continues to educate herself to the point where I believe she knows more than many "experts" about certain aspects of women's health. Kylee's courage and passion is nothing short of inspirational—and galvanizing.

The bottom line is this. Whether you are Alex's age, my mother's age, my wife's age, or anywhere in between, and whether you are currently in good health or are facing health issues, I know you will derive some benefit from *Hormone Basics*. I can say this because, while I may never have met you personally, I talk with women every single day with similar questions and concerns. So now I invite you to settle in and read the words on the following pages.

Learn. Ask questions. And always know there is hope.

2

What Do You Want & Why Aren't You Getting It?

To get what you want, you have to know what "it" is. That's why the first thing I'd like you to do is ask yourself what is really important in life. Is it how much money you make? How famous you are? What kind of education you get? If you've answered money, fame, family, love, health, job, location, religion, kids, pets, or relationships, you can count yourself among the masses who would probably answer in similar ways. And don't get me wrong; they're all reasonable answers.

After you've taken a few moments to answer the question of what's important, it's time to ask yourself how you'd prioritize these things in your life that you've identified. Do they all rate the same on your list of "needs"? Will you be devastated if you don't achieve fame as an actor, but only slightly disappointed if you don't get married or have children?

Certainly the idea of what has the most merit in our lives varies for each of us and are revised to one degree or another as we progress through life. This is true in part because the more we have a chance to really live life, the more things like relationships, family, love, and spirituality tend to increase in significance. But one of the most compelling contributors to everyone's overall quality of life—and the great equalizer for every single person on earth—is health status: how good we feel as we live our lives. For example, I think it's pretty common to under appreciate just how much our health affects every aspect of life until or unless something happens to remind us. True quality of life cannot be defined by all the "things" we have for one simple reason: things cease to matter altogether if we lose our good health. Obviously if we are sick or in pain, buying a fancier car or a bigger house won't cure us or make us happy.

If you ever have the opportunity to talk with people who know their time on earth is limited, I suspect they might tell you that good health, faith, and meaningful relationships are what they value the most. On the other hand, I would be surprised if they said that they had regrets about not having a classier car, a house in a certain neighborhood, or enough designer clothes. Of course, like I said, it is up to us to decide for ourselves what determines our own true quality of life. If we are lacking in healthy relationships, for example, does the life we are living have the kind of quality we want? If we are in poor physical health, is it possible to create or maintain positive, healthy relationships?

How hormones affect both physical and mental health and therefore the quality of life and wellbeing of women (and men) everywhere is a critical topic that demands our attention on a global scale. Because, while it is true that there is plenty of discussion about the topic of hormones, research and discussion has been much too focused on the symptoms of monthly cycles, menopause, and hormone replacement therapy.

Although knowledge alone is not power, all women would do well to learn as much as they can about what is happening in and to their bodies, especially in terms of the major role that hormones play. Too many women are suffering because they don't understand how their mental and physical health is being affected and what they can do to change the paradigm. Health is not something that affects only the individual either. Our good health, or lack of it, has a significant effect on the people around us: our spouses, boyfriends, girlfriends, parents, and coworkers. Sons, husbands, and dads (me included) all know how much the subject of hormones and their effect on women scares the living daylights out of us men. Why? Because most men know even less than women about the topic of hormones, let alone really understand what little they might have heard. More importantly, men feel uncomfortable because they know that whatever isn't "right" is not something they, as males, can fix or control.

Men fix things

Most people would agree that by nature men tend to be fixers. But if men are such fixers (and we are) and if men are the ones who have controlled most of the work in the medical field for centuries (and we are), exactly why haven't we made a conscious effort to try to "fix" the hormone challenge and the multitude of other problems that keep women suffering? Why exactly hasn't more research been undertaken in this field to help those in the 14 to 44 "forgotten" group? If you ask me, this disinterest could be one of the reasons things are so messed up. With that said, if the man in your life isn't qualified but is still trying to fix the "problem" related to your hormones, he is fighting a losing battle. And more likely than not his tendency to fix it—or you—will only make the situation worse.

I myself come from a long line of fixers. My dad is a fixer and I was, too—until I learned that being a fixer usually does more harm than good. I have learned that it's okay to want to try to help, but that it's better to do it from another perspective. I think the world would be an easier place to live if fixers underwent a basic transformation where they became "be-ers" instead. Fixers can learn how to just "be" by listening actively and attentively so they remain calm, empathetic, sympathetic, helpful, loving, and open—whether they fully understand the situation or not. So, my advice to fixers? *Just be.* It's a great approach that works wonders.

Men: If you feel a compulsion to fix, I hope you soon understand that one of the most crucial factors related to the health of the women in your life and the health of your relationships is that you stop trying to fix whatever it is you think is broken. It probably won't work and you probably aren't helping!

Okay, ladies, now it's your turn. Please try to understand that for every time and for whatever reason the man (or men) in your life may be aggravating, infuriating, or less than empathetic in regards to your hormones or "cycles," it is probably because he wants you to feel better. This means he will continue to feel bad as long as he thinks there is a problem and as long as you feel bad. In my humble opinion, all any of us want is to feel good and be happy. The men in your life should want you to feel good and be happy, too. It doesn't matter who they are—fathers, sons, brothers, husbands, or friends. If they don't, then you probably won't, and if that's the case then you need to seriously question the quality of any relationship where the other person doesn't want you to feel good and be happy.

The reality is that life throws us all curves from time to time and we all have things we might want to change. Big or small, we handle them the best way we know how. But while we're handling them, we often expect them to have as much impact on other people as they have on us. Well, I hate to break it to you, but this is not always the case. However dramatic, traumatic, horrible, critical, or momentous these challenges are or appear to be, they are OUR problems to sort out, even if we have help doing it. Problems always seem worse when they are ours—because they *are* ours! They never seem as serious or as stress-inducing to anyone else. We are all guilty of this misconception, but in the end, no matter how sad, frustrated, or angry you are, you'll never be sad, frustrated, or angry enough to make anyone else feel exactly the way you do.

The point? We all deserve a life of great quality—and it is up to us to try to figure out what that means and how to achieve it.

3

The Forgotten Hormone Years

Many of you have been inspired to read this book for a couple of reasons: (1) you want to know why you feel the way you do and (2) you want to know if hormones are the culprits and if they are, what to do about it. For those of you who are still asking, "Why should I care?" please know that it is to *all* of you that I direct my attention.

The best place to start is by letting you know that even if you think you're clueless about all things hormonal, you probably know more than you think you do.

For me personally, though, there's a reason I know what I do on the subject of hormones. It isn't only because I'm concerned for women, because I've read a few books on the subject, or even because I took a few courses on obstetrics and gynecology in chiropractic school. In fact, there's a much simpler explanation. It's because at one point in my life I too suffered from symptoms that were confusing, frightening, and completely unnerving. Some of them might be the same kinds of symptoms you are suffering from right now. In fact, even though my symptoms were hugely alarming, in a great feat of denial I chose to ignore them—until the time came that they threatened to destroy my health forever. You'll be hearing more about that story later, the one about how my hormones and my health were locked in a fight that almost cost me my life. Suffice it to say that it's clear to me that if it weren't for what happened to me then, I might never have become so committed to learning what I needed to know. And if I had never gotten the answers I needed, I would not be able to share them with you now.

Let's start with the premise of *Hormone Basics*: that there isn't anything that happens inside your body that isn't in some way related to your hormones. If we accept this is true, then we need to look at the ways in which hormones can affect you at any stage of your life so you can begin to see how relevant they are to your overall health. The next section lists the most common symptoms and conditions associated with the ways hormones function in the human body, specifically targeting things that can happen when hormones get out of whack. When we say hormone levels are "out of whack," we simply mean they aren't balanced as they should be to keep the body functioning normally. When you look at this list you might be surprised to find that you could be suffering from one sort or another of hormonal imbalance, even if it's a minor one. You will also see that the list is long. Believe it or not, many other symptoms and side effects of hormonal imbalance have *not* been included because such an extensive list could fill an entire book all by itself.

Symptoms and/or conditions of hormonal imbalance include:

Depression, mood swings, anger, agitation, irritability, emotional hypersensitivity, increased stress, lack of attentiveness and concentration; inability of body to meet conditions of stress; headaches/migraines; food cravings; acne; increased body fat (especially in the hips, abdomen, and thighs); painful, abnormal periods (dysmenorrhea; irregular periods; oligomenorrhea (infrequent periods) and amenorrhea (absence of periods); decreased energy and stamina;

water retention; PMS; breast tenderness, enlargement, lumps, uterine fibroids, PCOS (Polycystic Ovary Syndrome), cysts; fibromyalgia; salt and water imbalance (muscle problems, uterine contraction (cramps); decreased resistance to disease (weakened immune system); carbohydrate/metabolism imbalances (weight gain/loss); lack of ambition/motivation; increased pain perception; development of sexual characteristics; increased or decreased libido (sex drive); sleep problems (insomnia, fatigue); decreased brain functioning, loss of memory; imbalanced HDL/LDL levels; prevention of cholesterol deposits or plaque that can lead to heart attacks and strokes; promotion of cell growth, especially of uterine lining and breast tissue; bone growth and strength, halting of growth of long bones (begins at puberty); stimulation to maturity of egg-containing follicle in ovaries; development of fetal brain and nervous system; maintenance of lining of blood vessels; blood pressure levels; promotion of normal cell life cycles; red blood cell levels; cortisol levels; gall bladder function; back health and conditions; fertility/infertility; hand-to-eye coordination; muscle toning/building; expansion of blood vessels; factors that contribute to hardening of the arteries; tissue hydration; body temperature regulation, including hot flashes and night sweats; bladder infections; incontinence, urinary frequency; vaginal dryness; *candida* (yeast) infections; decreased breast size; cold hands and feet; constipation/diarrhea; heavy bleeding, clotting; dry eyes, sinus conditions; autoimmune disorders, such as Irritable Bowl Syndrome, Crohn's Disease, Leaky Gut Syndrome, rheumatoid arthritis, osteoporosis, endometriosis (uterine lining condition); cardiovascular disease; wrinkles; thyroid levels; blood sugar and insulin levels; breast, endometrial, uterine cancer; and copper toxicity.

Do you find this list, partial as it is, as mind-boggling as I do? Do you see a number of symptoms or conditions that might apply to you—and that you now know can be caused by some kind of hormone imbalance? If the answer to that question is yes, it's the perfect starting point for our discussion on what hormones are and do. Remember, if you do find some of your challenges on this list, the important thing is not to get discouraged. Instead, use what you are learning to feel encouraged. Because the more you know about your hormones the more you will know about how to better manage them. And managing your hormones effectively means taking back and keeping control of your life.

What are hormones?

Since we are keeping this basic, we won't attempt to learn all there is to know about the more than 50 hormones that researchers have identified in the human body. If you're interested and motivated you can research those on your own in the future (something I highly recommend). After we learn the basics about hormones, we will also discuss stress and how it is directly linked to all things hormonal.

Hormones are made of molecules, as is all life. The *Merriam Webster Dictionary* defines a molecule as "the smallest particle of a substance." Not all molecules are created equal, however. Some are much more potent than others and hormones, it turns out, are *very* potent molecules indeed. To understand just how powerful hormones are, it helps to know that it usually takes as little as a *billionth of a gram* of a hormone for it to do its job. To help you visualize how minute such a hormone particle would be, picture a grain of salt. Now picture that grain of salt with the approximately 120,000 hormones that can fit inside of it. It helps me to think of a hormone as a very, very tiny, but incredibly powerful bubble.

Grain of salt compared to a hormone.

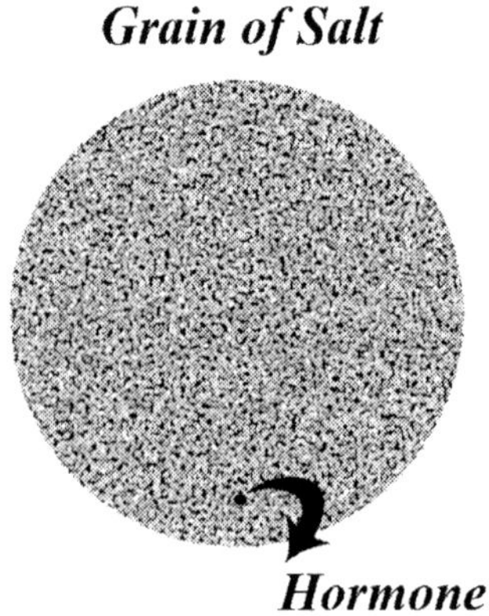

These days there's quite a bit of talk about hormones. Unfortunately, a lot of what's being said is wrapped in a cloud of negativity. When most people talk about hormones it is in the context of comments like these—and always accompanied by groans of despair: "It's that time of the month"; "I gained all this weight"; "I'm feeling so bloated"; "I don't have any energy"; or "She's such a witch today; it's probably PMS." I'd be surprised if you don't hear things like this pretty regularly and if you don't say them yourself from time to time.

There's some good news and not-so-good news here, so let's take the not-so-good news first. Hormones *are* playing a role in every weird, painful, uncomfortable, life altering, and possibly health jeopardizing feeling or condition you are experiencing or that you have experienced at some time or another. Therefore, the hormone "excuse" is not and has never been an excuse at all. But if you don't understand how or why hormones are affecting you, you can't do anything to help yourself. Furthermore, if you are under the horrible misconception that you can control hormones "on your own," or that it is up to you to "handle them," the way some people seem to think you should, you can let yourself off the hook right now. You are not a thermostat that runs hot and cold and that can be set to perform higher or lower upon demand. It's not that easy. Additionally, even if up until now you knew you needed help or had questions, it's likely you had no idea where to go to get those questions answered.

Just refer back to the list of common symptoms and conditions associated with hormone imbalances on pages 30 and 31 for evidence that hormones may indeed be the reason for any number of conditions, symptoms, or feelings you and your body are experiencing.

Of course the good news is that this is not the way it has to be.

We'll get into that part of the equation a little later on, though. For now, let's get back to hormones and what they do.

How hormones communicate

The tiny but powerful hormone "bubbles" described above have the extremely important task of carrying messages to and from all parts of the body. When everything is working right—in other words, when all our bodily parts are working as they should, both individually and in sync with all the other parts—both the body and brain remain in balance. When they are in balance, you stay healthy. And when your body and brain are healthy and in balance, you feel absolutely great!

It might be a good time to take a minute to take stock of how you feel right now. Do you feel wide awake, energized, tired, sad, achy, excited, or angry? Are you in a gigantic funk? Maybe you feel like throwing something. Whatever you feel, it's important to ask yourself whether the things you are feeling are, as you may have been told before, "all in your head." Of course, depending on your perspective, they always are—sort of. But a truer statement would be that what you feel is "all in your brain" because your brain is your body's command center. The brain makes everything happen; it starts, ends, and controls the way everything works—or doesn't work, as the case may be. Finally, critically, the brain is where pain, discomfort, and all other sensations originate.

One of the ways your brain communicates with every other part of your body is through the nervous system. I'll give you an example. You may have heard stories about people who have had an arm or leg amputated and who, even after the limb has been removed, report having continued sensations like itching, pain, and numbness in the arm, hand, leg, or foot that is no longer there. Unbelievable as it seems, these individuals actually feel these sensations keenly even though the limb is gone. This phenomenon is referred to as "phantom pain." How is this possible? Again, it all starts in the brain, which sends impulses to every other part of the body.

In other words, every sensation we experience, whether it is pressure, pain, numbness, itching, hot, or cold, is processed first in the brain and then sent from the brain in the form of a signal back to that part of the body where the sensation originated. The brain is trying to let you know what is taking place, where it is taking place, and if something needs to be done about it. And this is only one of the countless amazing ways our bodies function.

In essence, the brain is constantly receiving and sending messages—infinite numbers of messages—to the rest of the body, similarly to how you might send emails or text messages to a friend. The body sends a message just the way you send a message in that you naturally expect that message will travel to reach the desired recipient, in this case via the Internet. Occasionally, however, the system breaks down. Anyone who has ever used a computer or cell phone knows how frustrating it is when service goes down and the connection is broken. Sometimes you're in a dead zone where there is no service or maybe the connection is bad and you can't hear the other person; sometimes your message doesn't make it through or sometimes only part of it goes through, leaving your attachments behind in the black hole of cyberspace. What is the cause of these disruptions? *Interference.*

Of course the body doesn't use the Internet to communicate, but it works in a similar fashion to send our messages out to the right places via its own version of a communication system, called the *nervous system*. The nervous system can be compared to the phone lines through which the Internet operates, with a series of thousands upon thousands of little lines that connect everything in the body to make it one big system. The "computer" that houses and directs this amazingly complex communication system is nothing other than the brain.

The nervous system is responsible for speeding the brain's directives wherever they are meant to go. It is comprised of bundles of nerves and these nerves serve to make the necessary connections between the directives and their intended recipients. The biggest of these bundles forms your *spinal cord*. The spinal cord, which attaches to the bottom of the brain, is the mechanism through which all the messages sent and received by the brain travel. In other words, the brain communicates its messages to all other parts of the body through the spinal cord and the brain receives messages that travel back through the nerves of the spinal cord to let it know how everything is or is not working. Your spinal cord is tucked safely away within the bones, or vertebra, of the spinal column to help protect this information "super highway." The spinal cord has 31 pairs of spinal nerves that emanate outwards from in between each vertebra like branches on a tree and then continue to branch off until they have reached every part of the body. This obviously includes the brain and the parts of your body that affect and control your hormones.

It might help to picture your brain and nervous system as an upside-down tree. Your brain is represented by the thick, ball-like roots of the tree; your spinal cord is represented by the tree trunk; your nerves are represented by all the branches; and your muscles, skin, organs, and so on, by the leaves.

The Central Nervous System (or CNS).

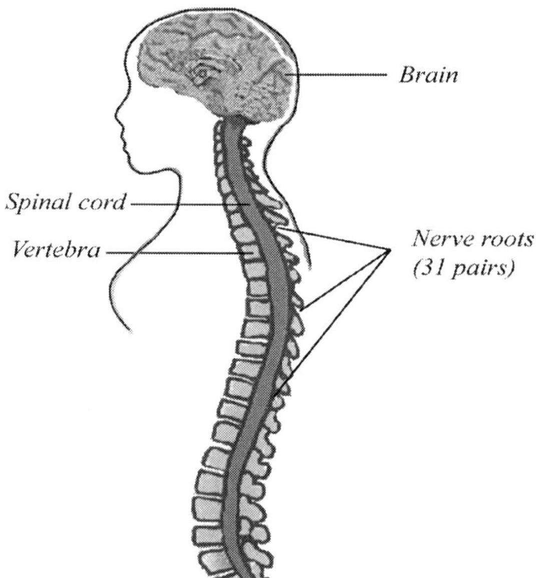

Again, it almost goes without saying that the way your brain and nerves interact with your hormones is an incredibly complex process, but remember, we don't need to know everything there is to know. We only need to know enough to understand how it affects *us right now*. With that in mind, if we look at the "branches on our tree"—in other words, the nerves of our spinal cord—we see that one of their destinations is the system of the body known as the *endocrine system*. The endocrine system is another complex system, but this one contains the *glands* that produce—that's right!—our hormones.

The endocrine system is like the nervous system in that it helps control all the processes and activities in the body. These systems are "booted up" long before you are actually born and will continue working until you die. The hormones produced at conception and prior to birth made sure your spinal cord, brain, and entire nervous system formed correctly. The endocrine system makes sure you develop the way you should in order for your *reproductive system* (which includes the ovaries, uterus, and breasts) to mature appropriately and for your immune system to keep you healthy. In addition, the endocrine system controls blood-sugar (glucose) and insulin levels, something we'll talk about later, as well as your *metabolism*, a term used to describe how your body stores and uses energy. These are just a few of the many tasks the endocrine system controls.

It is your nervous system that works with the endocrine and reproductive systems to produce the hormones the body needs for controlling its internal functions. The number of hormones produced by these systems and whether the systems work properly depends on many things. One factor is the nature of the signal received by the brain, which is then sent out to the rest of the body, and then sent back to the brain again. This is where chiropractic care can be so beneficial to your health because it assesses how much interference there may be when a hard bone (vertebra) puts pressure on the soft nerves and then helps correct the problem with a gentle adjustment of the bone. This adjustment affects whatever the nerves control, like hormones, muscle, organs, and the immune system.

Hormones are not produced solely by the reproductive and endocrine systems, however. They are also made in other areas of the body, such as in the skin and in fat cells. In these areas, hormones are produced in relatively small amounts—unless you have more fat cells than you should. Having too many fat cells is something that can be problematic as well. You will understand why a little later in your reading.

Now that you have a better understanding of how your tiny, but powerful hormone "bubbles" work, the next thing on the agenda is to understand their composition.

4

Hormones & Nutrients

Short of a biochemistry lecture, the absolute simplest way to describe the makeup of a hormone is to say that it is made from *amino acids*, *cholesterol*, and *nutrients*.

There are more than 100 amino acids that occur in nature, 20 of which can form proteins. Proteins have many functions. For example, they are an essential part of the immune (protection) system, they form the body's muscles, and transport oxygen. Amino acids, which are essential to every form of life, are a huge part of the body's nutritional foundation. Humans produce 10 of the 20 protein-forming amino acids on their own, but the others must be supplied through the food we eat. Failure to obtain enough of even one of the 10 essential amino acids, those that we cannot make ourselves, results in degradation of the body's proteins—muscle and so forth—to obtain that one amino acid that is needed. Unlike fat and starch, the human body does not store excess amino acids for later use; therefore, amino acids must be replenished through the food we eat every day.

You may be surprised to learn that the second and even more important element in a hormone's makeup is cholesterol. Cholesterol often gets a bad rap because it's linked to LDL, or low-density lipoprotein—the "bad" cholesterol, and too much bad cholesterol can lead to heart attacks and stroke. But you may also be surprised to learn that cholesterol has a number of health benefits, including its ability to help the body form the vitamin that comes from exposure to the sun, vitamin D (the benefits of which will be discussed later). But before you start chomping on those cheese fries or that burger, you might want to take a closer look at whether you might be getting too much of a good thing.

Cholesterol

Cholesterol is a waxy substance produced by the liver, the organ we rely on to process toxicity from the body. Cholesterol is found in certain foods and required for the production of hormones. It also builds cell walls and helps us digest fat. Because our liver automatically produces about 1,000 milligrams of cholesterol a day, we definitely don't need to add to it through the foods we eat. Of course that would mean never eating another French fry, so maybe not. But it's hard to avoid cholesterol entirely because so many foods contain it. Just to give you some idea, cholesterol is found in all foods that come from animal sources, like eggs, meat, and whole-fat dairy products (milk, cheese, ice cream, and so on). These foods are loaded with cholesterol, whereas vegetables, fruits, and grains contain none at all. That's right. Nada, zilch, zip.

Nutritional sources, or nutrients, are the other close relatives of hormones. Most of us know by now that it is the nutrient content of foods like fruits, vegetables, nuts, and seeds that makes them good for us in their capacity to keep us healthy and help us grow and function normally. Some nutrients can be produced inside the body; others are referred to as *essential nutrients* because they are essential to our body's survival. We can only get essential nutrients through two sources: the foods we eat or nutritional supplements. As you can see from the illustration below, nutrients are even smaller than hormones. It is when many nutrient "bubbles" band together that they form a hormone.

Since the nutrients in the things you eat and drink are a big part of what makes up your hormones, it naturally follows that your hormones can only be as helpful and healthy as what you eat.

Nutrient compared to a hormone.

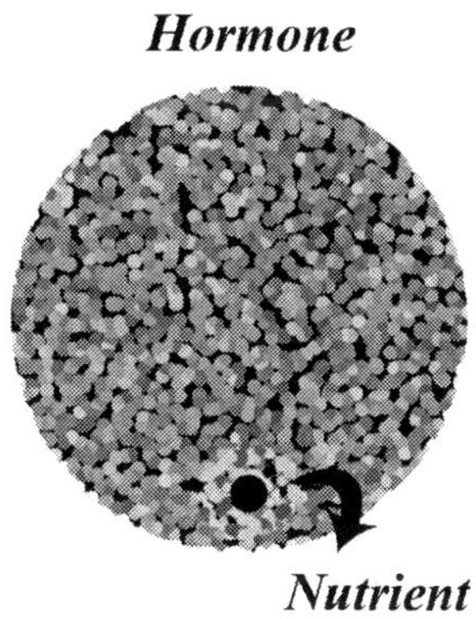

There are other things that contribute to helping you feel your best, but giving your body the best nourishment you can is a great start.

There is a saying you may have heard that originally started in the computer business: "Garbage in, garbage out." This, of course, is true for many aspects of life. For example, you are only going to get out of something what you put in to it, whether it's life in general, how hard you work at your chosen career, or one of the best examples: the food you put into your body. What you ingest has a direct and substantial effect on how the status of your health and on how you feel every day.

A good example of getting the results you want might be baking a cake. If you are baking a chocolate cake and you leave out some of the necessary ingredients—like chocolate—or substitute one item for another—like water for milk—your cake won't come out as it was intended. If you use corn meal instead of flour, or perhaps reverse the indicated amounts of sugar and salt, a dramatically different cake (and likely a very disappointing cake) will be the result. What comes out of the oven might still resemble what you expected your cake to look like, but in quality and taste you can be sure it would fall far short.

In terms of what you eat on a daily basis, if most of it comes from a drive-through, a box, a bag, or a Styrofoam cup, if it needs to be heated in the microwave, or if it can be "super-sized," chances are you aren't getting many of the nutrients required for your body to work correctly and keep working correctly. Our bodies are created to take in wholesome foods that are as close to their original, natural state as possible in order to function most effectively and efficiently. This includes eating them without overcooking them—or without cooking them at all.

Ideally, organic fruits, vegetables, nuts, and seeds are best for your body. Together with reasonable amounts of lean meat, such as fish or chicken that is either wild-caught, organic, or natural (with no added hormones or antibiotics), they will give your body the best chance to get the nutrients it needs without all the other junk we so often add. Avoid frying and overcooking what you eat and you will also increase your chances of getting the most nutritional value out of whatever it is that you put in your body.

If eating fresh fruits and vegetables is a challenge for you, a good option is to buy and eat them in their frozen form. Frozen fruits and vegetables keep longer than fresh, first of all, and second, they often retain a high concentration of their nutritional value because most are frozen almost immediately after they are harvested. For many people, locating, buying, and eating organic food may not be practical or cost-effective. My advice is to do the best you can as often as you can. Don't forget that there is always something you can do to improve your health through the foods you eat. For a few excellent resources on organic products and eating well, check out our website, www.hormonebasics.com.

The SAD American Diet

Sadly, many people eat considerably less fruit and fewer vegetables, nuts, and grains than are recommended by scientists. There are lots of reasons for their food choices, but most blame hectic schedules, lack of convenience, and cost. The unfortunate reality is that far too many Americans are on what's called the Standard American Diet, or SAD. This is a very "sad" fact and one that may be at the core of the poor state of our collective health. How closely does the following daily menu from the SAD diet below describe *your* eating habits?

The (very) SAD American Diet

For breakfast you eat one or more of the following: white toast, bagel, doughnut, or croissant; cereal (a variety with added sugar); an item from a drive-through, such as a latte, mocha, or another high-sugar coffee drink; an "energy" drink or caffeinated soda.

For your mid-morning snack (a must-have, since you are probably starving or crashing because breakfast has left you empty and nutritiously unfortified), you eat something from the vending machine (processed and lacking any real nutritional value), a leftover doughnut or whatever else you can get your hands on, an energy drink, soft drink, or coffee drink to perk you up.

For lunch you eat some kind of fast food, perhaps a burger, fries, pizza, tacos, burritos, or fried chicken. Oh, and don't forget the soft drink.

For your mid-afternoon snack (which you again desperately need because you're crashing again), you eat one or more of the following: a candy bar or other sweet treat and perhaps a caffeinated soda or coffee drink.

For dinner you eat something you heat in the box or bag it came in, such as a hamburger, fries, pizza, tacos, burritos, fried chicken, Chinese food, pasta, or wings, plus a soft drink, or possibly alcohol (if you are of legal drinking age).

If this menu seems familiar, you are probably eating the SAD diet pretty consistently. And you are not alone! Most people who eat this way generally eat very few fruits and vegetables. Yes, the Big Mac may have a lettuce leaf on it and ketchup is made from tomatoes, but that doesn't begin to get you the nutrients your body needs. Even if there *are* vegetables somewhere in the food products you regularly consume, they're likely so overcooked and so over-processed that most of their vitamin and mineral content has effectively gone straight down the drain. It is indeed a SAD fact that the majority of what many Americans eat undergoes so much processing that by the time the food gets to them it has been entirely stripped of its nutritional value. That sliver of lettuce or glimpse of a pickle in between the bleached white bun or garnishing the plate next to all the other stuff just doesn't do the trick.

Skipping meals

Skipping meals is another American habit that backfires on health and wellbeing—with the possible exception being that you were only going to fill your body with garbage anyway. This type of eating pattern affects more than just our hormones. There are those who don't eat breakfast because they "don't have time," and those who skip lunch for the same reason; or perhaps they're trying to eat less or nothing at all to shed a few pounds. Unfortunately, people who don't eat breakfast are probably starving by lunchtime (if they haven't gorged themselves on sweets mid-morning). Because they're so hungry when they finally sit down to eat, they have a tendency to overeat, shoving more food than they need into their body so quickly that by the time their body realizes it's full it is actually over capacity and they are left with a stuffed and bloated feeling. And that's just the beginning, because another crash is soon to follow.

The worst of the bad eating habits may be committed by those who only eat one meal a day at the end of the day. Meals like this tend to be of poor nutritional value and consumed in large amounts to compensate for the lack of food eaten the rest of the day. This means eating more than they need and more than they should when they finally do have a meal. Furthermore, most people decrease their activity late in the day. A few hours sitting at the computer or in front of the television after a big meal is not the type of physical activity required to stimulate the digestive processes and late-eaters end up going to bed with a large portion of the evening meal still stuck in their digestive tract. Did you know that what your body doesn't properly break down and expel actually rots inside of you? That's right, stuck inside the body food quickly decays, becoming rancid and toxic to the system. Pretty gross, right?

Many of us suffer under the misconception that we can benefit from sporadic eating habits because we aren't eating as much food overall on any given day. But this is a fallacy. Such eating habits more often contribute to poor health, including lack of weight loss—or even weight gain. And if your eating habits are inconsistent, your metabolism—the way your body burns food and produces and expends energy—will more than likely be inconsistent as well. Over time your confused metabolism tricks the brain and body into thinking it is experiencing a form of starvation. When this happens, the body and brain attempts to store anything you put into it for future use. Because the body's mechanism for storage is in our fat (cholesterol), you can see how eating inconsistently or less often than the body requires is not necessarily the way to lose what you may consider "excess" fat.

The reality is that your body needs to be fed on a regular basis to work most efficiently. I encourage my patients to eat small amounts about every 3 to 4 hours. This usually limits the amounts of what they eat because they aren't as hungry; plus it helps keep the body's metabolism working consistently, and that helps burn fat. When you eat the right things in the correct amounts you will find you establish an essential foundation for achieving and maintaining optimal health.

If you're wondering how it's possible to take the time to eat 3 healthy meals a day—let alone 6 or 7 smaller ones—with the hectic schedules most of us have and short of hiring a personal chef, I'll share some of my secrets with you. And after learning how you can prepare healthy food easily, I expect you to feel at least a little guilty if you don't take advantage of the information.

Snacking tips

Here are a few quick and easy snacking alternatives to the vending machine or drive-through. On Sunday, boil a dozen eggs, but don't peel them. Put them back into the carton and mark it "hard-boiled." In the morning there's nothing simpler than taking one out, peeling it, and putting it aside either for some quick protein at breakfast or as an easy pick-me-up mid-morning or mid-afternoon. Eggs come in their very own convenient natural packaging and are great at satisfying cravings and to keep from "crashing" between meals.

Fruits, nuts, and seeds also come in their own personal wrappers and are really the "no-excuse" snack. Throw a banana, orange, apple, or a handful of pistachios into your purse, briefcase, or cup-holder and you've got the perfect snack to zap your hunger or need to nibble. They don't take up much room either. I've been known to carry a handful of nuts in my pocket if I don't have a better way to keep them with me and I figure any lint just adds fiber. Grapes are another great option, and if you really want to get crazy, freeze them the way our family does. It's a totally different snacking experience. I do the same with bananas. Alex and I have grown to prefer frozen bananas over fresh ones and because overripe bananas can often be found at a discounted price at the market they're perfect for freezing and for the pocketbook. The only way nuts and seeds are difficult to pack and eat is if you don't buy them. A small handful is an adequate serving, too, so they take up very little space as well.

Another suggestion is to take advantage of a quiet Sunday to prepare raw vegetables for the entire week. Vegetables like broccoli, cauliflower, carrots, cucumbers, peppers, and celery make wholesome, crunchy, bite-sized snacks and can be stored in the frig for days. Grabbing a handful or two of fresh veggies on your way out the door is easy and practical—and can save you from yourself later on when the only thing within reach is the office doughnut box or school vending machines.

These are just a few ways to eat healthier with little to no effort or extra cost. In fact, these types of options are ordinarily much cheaper than fast food and the garbage housed in machines.

Speaking of health, you may not be aware that although the United States is usually one of the world's top two spenders in total "health care" expenditures, we Americans fall far, far below most of the other countries in the world with regard to our actual health. That's an interesting statement about the way we take care of ourselves—or don't. Furthermore, for the first time in history children's life spans are projected to be shorter than that of their parents! That means if parents are expected to live into their late 70s or 80s, their kids are now only expected to only live into their 60s or 70s. If you are young now, this may not seem all that critical, but I can guarantee it will matter a lot as you age. Think about what that implies about your health and what you eat.

Now, back to the "garbage in, garbage out" analogy and how it applies to your hormones and overall health. A diet consisting of fresh fruits, plenty of vegetables, nuts, seeds, chicken, turkey, fish, perhaps red meat (in small amounts), and plenty of water helps your hormones function to their best capacity. This helps you feel better and be healthier. If you exercise even half an hour every day, you will feel even better. In other words: healthy food = healthy hormones = a healthy you.

Most patients who come into our clinic for the first time tell me they have long forgotten what it's like to feel decent, let alone good or great. Not feeling good for these people has become a habitual state, one that developed gradually, so gradually that it went unnoticed—but more often ignored—for days, months, or years. Then one day they woke up and realized that they hadn't felt good for a long time and that it wasn't okay anymore. Most days they wake up tired, often with no more energy than when they went to bed. These people report gaining more weight than they lose, even if they diet. They feel tense and crabby more often than they feel happy, have more aches and pains and have them more often, and notice their skin isn't as smooth and soft as it used to be. Do any of these symptoms—or any from our long list—sound like you?

These circumstances are often in addition to any clinical conditions the patients have, like diabetes, high blood pressure, high cholesterol, or Irritable Bowel Syndrome. Sadly enough, much of the population in this country can identify with one or more of these medical challenges. The vast majority doesn't remember what it feels like to feel good or to be truly healthy. And if you don't feel good and you aren't healthy, how much fun can the rest of your life be?

5

Your Health & Hormones

Fortunately, you can change how you feel.

The best way to start is to figure out what it means to *you* to be "healthy." Does it mean the absence of feeling bad? Does it mean not having any particular symptoms that are serious enough to go to the doctor? Does it mean not having one or more diseases or conditions, such as diabetes, cancer, high cholesterol, irritable bowel, or high blood pressure, that end up forcing you to change the way you live your life?

Obviously, health means different things to different people. But I hope you understand that being healthy usually means more than just feeling good. Unfortunately, most of us don't know that we have health problems until it is too late.

For example, did you know that studies show that the first symptom in over half of all heart attacks is death? That means the victims didn't have any warning and because they had no warning (or did not recognize potential symptoms for what they really were), they never had the opportunity to take the necessary steps (seeing their doctor, for instance) to avert disaster. Without some of the "typical" signs that something is amiss, such as the loss of appetite, unexplained jaw pain, extreme fatigue, tightness in the chest, numbness down the left arm, or indigestion, many people have no idea they are in trouble. And don't think heart attacks are mostly a concern for just us males; the last time I checked the research showed that heart attacks still kill twice as many women as all cancers combined! It turns out that hormone imbalance and some of the methods for treating these imbalances are two important things that can affect the health of your heart and the health of your cardiovascular system.

Now back to the question of how to define health. According to Webster's *New World Dictionary*, *health* is "physical and mental well-being; freedom from disease, pain, or defect; normality of physical and mental functions." What this means is that being healthy is a state where the body *and* the brain work properly and feel good. Human beings were not created to experience disease or to be sick. Our hormones should never be so out of balance that they make us unable to function normally. We should not hurt without undue cause either; not physically, as with headaches, backaches, or stomachaches, or emotionally, when there is no specific circumstance that is triggering our pain. When we do feel any of these things or experience pain that cannot be explained by a particular event, the one thing we can know for sure is that it is a symptom that something is wrong and that something greater is happening. That means whatever it is needs to be addressed before it gets any more severe.

Patients often ask me, "How did this happen? How did I get into this condition?" I share my theory with them that I believe we were created to be perfect beings; that we were born to be healthy and happy, not to be sick, diseased, or to live in pain. It's yet another unfortunate reality that though we may have been created to be perfect, we are the ones who mess things up. How? By living in an imperfect world! So, what matters is *how* we choose to live the life we have in the world we have been given. If we are more reactive than proactive we end up with the "garbage out" effect. This means if you don't take appropriate care of yourself by eating right, getting plenty of sleep and exercise, and keeping your stress levels low you won't feel as good and be as healthy as you can be or would like to be.

If a lack of information is the reason you haven't been doing more for yourself and your health, then that's easy to fix simply by reading this book. If you have a question that isn't answered in here, on our website (www.hormonebasics.com), or anywhere else you've looked, contact me directly. I tell my patients that I'm always here to help any way I can and this is true for my readers as well. Just call me, email me, or stop into the clinic, where you will always be welcome. My contact information is at the back of this book.

As I visit with people, I can see that they are often genuinely puzzled by how they've arrived at their current condition. Many times they are not really even sure how to describe what they feel. Many of them have no obvious family history for a major disease like cancer or heart disease. Many have never been diagnosed with any particular condition that would explain their symptoms. Many have never been in a major accident or even had a broken bone. What they do have in common is the feeling that something just isn't right. Of course, that feeling is the basis for what I think is the most common, undiagnosed, and untreated condition there is: *dis-ease.*

Dis-ease

Dis-ease comes from the word "disease," but the added hyphen changes its meaning considerably. *Disease* is an abnormal condition that impairs bodily functions and is associated with specific symptoms and signs. A disease may be caused by external factors like exposure to toxic substances (many of which you will find in your own home and will be discussed later in detail), a virus or bacteria, or by internal dysfunctions, such as cells that reproduce abnormally, autoimmune disease, or the inability of one of your organ systems to function as it should. By the time someone is diagnosed with a disease, he or she has probably already started seeing a health care provider. *Dis-ease*, on the other hand, is more about not being *at ease*;

that is, being uncomfortable, existing in a state that does not feel natural, one that may feel unhealthy or that may feel like a constant state of struggle as we talked about earlier on. Most of us struggle in life to some degree or another, but some of us do so much more than others. If you are living a life and lifestyle that is a struggle, one where you have to work at it just to survive, then you are living a life of dis-ease. And a prolonged lack of "ease" leads straight to *dis*-ease, something that often ultimately leads to full-blown "disease." The same is true for the state of stress, where too much stress leads to distress, or *dis*-stress. Not surprisingly, distress also tends to culminate in disease.

Recently I was visiting with a couple (we'll call them the "Wrights" to protect their identities) and their three kids. We were discussing this very topic of dis-ease. The Wrights are like most parents—and most people—who aren't aware that all of us have an event in common, an event that may have been so traumatic that we feel its effects for an entire lifetime. What is this event that each and every one of us has experienced? Yup: childbirth.

Clearly, childbirth is a process that none of us could have avoided. It is also a process that, simply by virtue of its traumatic nature, can set the stage for many potential problems later in life. Of course, you could argue the case that you have not experienced any noticeable ill effects from your own birth and that, if you happen to be a parent, neither have your children. You could argue that your children have been disease-free and that they have never had any significant illnesses or been in an accident. You could argue that without those kinds of life-changing events there is no evidence that you or they have experienced significant trauma. And to some degree you might be right. But you would be overlooking the fact that the process of being born is inherently a difficult one, even under the best of conditions. You probably don't remember it too well, of course, but leaving a warm, comfortable, secluded place (your mother's womb) to suddenly meet a bright white, loud, chaotic world could easily be the most intimidating and life-changing event of your life.

We may not remember how traumatized we might have been at the time, but numerous potential challenges present themselves as we are being born, at the very moment of and in the minutes after our birth. "Little things," such as the typical twisting of the head and neck past what would be considered a normal range of motion in order to aid in the delivery process or pulling of the body for the same reason. Although these techniques may be standard operating procedure during the delivery of a newborn, that doesn't mean the experience is any less formidable. Certainly, if we were to undergo the same kind of trauma later in life, at any age, we might well expect to experience severe pain and long-lasting repercussions from the injury. The only difference is that as a newborn we are relatively consciously unaware of our circumstances; as we get older we know when these things happen. Fortunately, babies' bodies are known for their flexibility because their bones are soft and forgiving. But the typical strain that the birthing process puts on a newborn can set the groundwork for future problems with the nervous system. These problems may not reveal themselves immediately—or even for years—but down the road symptoms will often appear with alarming consequences.

As big people we can complain, go to the doctor, or do whatever we feel is necessary to help us deal with our problem. But infants and toddlers really have only one way of letting us know they are uncomfortable or in pain: they cry. Some babies seem to cry a lot more than others, too. Apart from needing to be fed or have its diaper changed, why would that be? Quite possibly, babies that cry more than usual may still be recovering from their harsh entry into the world or from symptoms of an event that occurred shortly thereafter.

Here's an example. Some of the infants we treat in the clinic are brought in because they cry all the time. Their parents are tired, frustrated, and thoroughly worn to a frazzle by attempting to determine what's bothering their child. The baby is often in dire distress, trying to communicate its discomfort in the only way it knows how. Is it an allergy to formula or cow's milk, stomach problems, or just a bad disposition? It's hard to know. But if we approach the situation from the vantage point of the infant's birth trauma, we can look for associated trauma to the nervous system. If we determine the problem is nerve related, we then relieve the pressure on the affected nerves. Often, after the pressure on the nerves has been relieved, the baby shows an immediate shift in its constitution. Many times the excessive crying, called colic, ceases altogether before the baby has even left the clinic.

Miracles happen all around us if we are looking for them. Think of all the falls and resultant bumps on the head and tiny whiplashes infants and toddlers experience while learning to crawl and walk. As they get older the accidents don't stop, either; kids fall off bikes, on the ice, out of trees, and off balance beams; they tackle and get tackled in football, collide in soccer, and slide in baseball. All these tumbles cause physical imbalances in the system, and yet our children continue to develop right on schedule.

There are concerns, however. For instance, one more problem kids face today that wasn't in the mix when I grew up is all the time they spend at a computer and playing video games. Even before they reach school age, kids are sitting—or slouching—in a desk chair in front of a monitor, scrolling up and down and moving their heads over and over with the same motions over prolonged periods of time. The rest of us are all too familiar with the repetitive use of the mouse and keyboard and the stress it causes on our neck and shoulders, the toll it takes on our muscles and nerves. It's a wonder that any of us are still able to move! Thank goodness again that our bodies are so resilient and hardy.

But however resilient we are, all the little things that happen to us continue to add up. No one is exempt from how hard life can naturally be on a body over the course of time. It helps that babies and kids are naturally in tune with how they feel and that they will let us know—if we're listening. Unfortunately, as we grow into our teens and adulthood, we can lose the ability to sense problems at their inception. Maybe we're just too busy to notice or to recognize the warning signs until they are raging full force. We tend to ignore the original source of the problem and we ignore pain. Since pain is the body's way of letting us know that something is really wrong, I suggest that if you feel pain, you let somebody who can help you know about it.

Pain

It is true that pain manifests in numerous different ways. If you cut your finger with a knife you feel immediate pain and the source is easy to distinguish. But most of the aches and pains we experience, both physical and emotional, come from deep-rooted causes that may be much less obvious. They may not be due to a sudden accident or incident, but to multiple problems that have compiled over time. This is one reason it doesn't make sense to treat individual symptoms. Health care providers must look at the whole person and her symptoms in context in order to provide true, "healing" care. With that said, it can be challenging to pinpoint when your symptoms really started or when you began feeling less than your usual self. Either way, as most of us know, treating the symptoms usually results in only a temporary cure; the same symptoms soon return, often worse than before. It would be like a dentist trying to treat your horribly painful cavity by telling you to stop eating so much sugar and to brush more often, but not drilling and filling the cavity—or vice versa. In essence, neither approach alone would be enough to ensure the problem gets treated and preventative measures are taken so that similar conditions will not return.

Whether it is in regard to hormones, aches and pains, or any other type of ailment one statement I hear continually is, "I remember having this same problem years ago; it got better for a while, but it keeps coming back again and again." I wonder if these individuals really understand what they are telling me: that the source problem was never appropriately treated in the first place. So, whether they just ignored it or took a pill for the pain, it keeps returning over and over, usually with more of a vengeance. This process can repeat itself in an endless loop of pain and temporary release from the pain or proceed to the point where the symptoms become permanent fixtures in their lives.

Our bodies have their own way of dealing with problems. Sometimes they produce their own natural opiates, or painkillers, in response to an injury. This ability rises from the need for survival, and this can be one reason that the pain we experience improves for the time being, or even disappears altogether. In the days of the caveman and cave woman, our life depended on our ability to hunt, gather, and escape from our predators. If we were unlucky enough to suffer from pain of some kind to the point we couldn't do these things efficiently, we would be sure to perish.

When you start paying more attention to yourself and how you really feel, you will find you know when something doesn't feel right; these are ways in which your body and your brain are telling you that something needs your attention. Again, the sooner you catch the problem the easier it can be to fix it. Plus, from long experience I can tell you that getting into a better state of health is nothing more than a matter of committing to it and staying with it.

6

Carbohydrates, Sugars, Fats, & Their Effects

So far, we have discussed hormones, nutrients, and health, and that one way to help yourself enjoy better health—which includes the state of your hormones—is through your diet, the food you eat. *I am not talking about dieting*. Let me repeat that: I am not talking about any kind of a diet—at least not the way the word "diet" is used by most of our culture today. Instead, we need to think of our daily "diet" as an eating plan, one that addresses how the food we eat affects our hormones and our bodies. Can it really be that simple? Yes.

Carbohydrates

Since you now know your hormones are made from nutrients that come from what you eat, the next step is to talk about another important food element: *carbohydrates*. I know you've heard of carbohydrates, or "carbs," especially in the context of "low-carb" dieting. But I think most people are thoroughly confused about what a carbohydrate really is, because the term has been so overused and misused.

In reality, a carbohydrate is basically nothing more than an organic compound, or sugar, that the body absorbs and then changes into energy. We all need energy to keep us functioning and alive. If our bodies were cars, the carbohydrates would be the tiny bubbles of fuel they need to keep going.

Our blood is responsible for maintaining the levels of our sugars, or carbs, and keeping the levels balanced is critical for our overall health. Imbalances in sugar levels left unchecked for too long can result in "blood-sugar" conditions like diabetes.

So, here's the scoop on blood. As we discussed, the nervous and endocrine systems carry messages from the brain to the rest of the body and back to the brain again. Blood is another way that these messages travel. Picture an interstate highway, perhaps like the ones in Los Angeles but with a million times more traffic. In this case, all the traffic that rushes up and down these superhighways—your blood vessels and arteries—are nutrients that come from the foods you eat, including sugars, water, and oxygen.

If your arteries and veins are the major highways, then your capillaries are the smaller roads or side streets. Your capillaries draw the blood away from our arteries so that the nutrients ultimately reach all the peripheral areas of the body, from the tips of your fingers to the end of your toes and to the top of your head.

Now let's return to the carbohydrates (sugars) that are flowing nonstop through the arteries and capillaries to provide the fuel we need for energy. Most of us know sugar as the granulated white stuff that looks like salt and goes in our coffee and in baked goods to pacify our sweet tooth. But if you've ever confused the two you know there's a big difference. This kind of white sugar or "table" sugar is called sucrose and comes from sugarcane plants. There are many other types of sugars, however. For example, glucose is made when the body breaks down starches and fructose is the sugar found naturally in fruits. There are also chemical, or artificial, sweeteners. These are manufactured products like Aspartame and Saccharin and should not be confused with natural sugars. The best sugars for the body are the ones that naturally come from fruits, grains, and vegetables. These are called "complex carbohydrate sugars" and are the ones our bodies and brains need and use most efficiently to produce energy and to keep our cells healthy.

You'll note that many natural sugars have the scientific ending of "ose," like fructose, sucrose, and lactose. But we can't assume that just because the word has "ose" on the end that it is a natural sugar—that is, from a natural source like a fruit or a vegetable. In fact, many chemical, or synthetic, sweetener manufacturers began tacking "ose" on at the end of their products' names to fool us into thinking they were also natural, but this is not the case at all. *These sweeteners do not break down in the body and do not contribute to the body's need for fuel.* The reality is that some of these sweeteners have been shown to cause cancer in laboratory tests and I assure you are in no way good for you. There are a couple of sources of natural sugars, such as Stevia and Xylitol, on the other hand, that are derived from plants and are easier for your body to break down and use than the artificial types prevalent in most sodas, so-called energy drinks, and most processed foods.

While it is important to know that the sweeteners used in the majority of foods you buy at the grocery store or eat in restaurants are much worse for you than the sugars that come from natural sources, it is the type and the amount of sugar you eat on a regular basis that is the biggest concern. The average person is unaware that the vast majority of foods we see on our grocery shelves are loaded with sugar of one kind or another. Ketchup, breads, mayonnaise, pasta sauce, salad dressing: most contain large amounts of sugar, often in the form of high-fructose corn syrup, one of the worst kinds of sweetener there is for the body. It is now estimated by the United States government that the average American consumes approximately 2 to 3 pounds of sugar every week. This equals between 100 and 150 pounds of sugar a year! Just 20 years ago Americans were eating only about a quarter of that amount, or 20 to 25 pounds a year. It is no wonder that obesity and all the other diseases related to excessive weight have also increased exponentially in children as well as in adults.

What this means is that when you get most of your carbohydrates from foods other than fruits, vegetables, and/or whole grains your body can't always use what it is taking in for energy the way it should. When the body can't use what it takes in or can't get rid of it appropriately it will respond by attempting to store what's left—in this case, the non-utilized carbs—as fat. What is even worse, however, is that because the incoming carbs are generally processed through the addition of more high-fat- and high-sugar-content foods, when they reach their resting place as stored fat they have all sorts of toxic material attached to them. A little later on we'll review some government tests that show just how dangerous this can be.

What fat isn't

And don't think health problems are confined to those who believe they're "fat." First of all, fat is a subjective term, as most of us can appreciate. More importantly, however, is the fact that fat is not inherently bad. We have given it a bad name, but *fat* is actually body tissue that does the critical job of storing the necessary energy we all need. So, no matter how skinny we might be, without stores of fat we would die. Technically, fat, or cholesterol, is actually the building block for all our hormones. That means that, at least in the correct amounts, fat is a very good—and very important—thing indeed.

Also, remember that being thin is not necessarily the same thing as being healthy. Whatever your body weight, if you aren't eating foods that provide you with the nutrients you need you will still be storing bad stuff—toxins—in whatever amount of body fat, however small, that you have. Skinny people aren't always healthy and heavier people aren't always sick. Whatever category you fit or wherever you fit in the spectrum, the thing that matters is that you aren't fooling yourself about your health.

If your body is not properly breaking down and then using or getting rid of the sugars you eat (that is, it is instead storing it in the form of fat and toxic buildup), it will not only make a difference in your weight but, equally as important, it will make a difference in your hormone levels, body shape, energy levels, mood, ability to concentrate, and more. If you continue to eat enough of the "bad" foods, the habit may eventually keep you from maintaining normal hormone levels over time. And by now you know that this can lead to diabetes, cholesterol imbalances, heart problems, high blood pressure, and yes, an increased risk for cancer.

There are two types of carbohydrates (remember, these are basically just sugars): complex, or unrefined, carbohydrates and refined carbohydrates.

Complex (unrefined) carbohydrates are those natural sugars that come from fruits, vegetables, whole grains, nuts, beans, and so on. They are broken down and absorbed more slowly in the body so they can be used more efficiently for energy. These types of sugars contribute to happy hormones and healthy bodies.

Refined carbohydrates are found in table sugar (sucrose), corn syrup, and high-fructose corn syrup, in all other refined and processed sugars, and in foods like breads, cakes, pasta, candy, soda, bagels, doughnuts, and pizza. Some might say they're in all the stuff that tastes good, but if these are the sources on which your body and hormones rely for energy, it will be sorely disappointed.

7

The "Skinny" on Insulin & Fat

Sugar levels in the blood, a result of what we eat, control a very important chemical we must have to live and be healthy. This chemical, called *insulin*, may be familiar to you if you know someone with diabetes. Diabetes is much more common today than it used to be, what with the ever-increasingly higher amounts of sugar (and processed foods) our society consumes. In fact, there is a good chance you may yourself be diabetic or have a family member who is, since 23.6 million people in the United States —8% of the population— have it. Because diabetes is now so common, many people don't realize how serious and potentially deadly a disease it is. If left untreated or poorly managed, diabetes can cause eventual blindness, amputation of one or more limbs, and death. Insulin and blood sugar levels are therefore of grave concern for diabetics, but they are also important for everyone else.

Insulin

Insulin is the chemical that helps the sugar get from your blood into your cells for energy. Think of insulin as a little taxicab. Without enough insulin taxis, the sugars get left at the curb (stored in your body as fat) and aren't able to get to where they belong to be used for energy. The good sugars (complex/unrefined carbohydrates) allow your body to make just enough insulin to get the sugar into your cells; because there is very little leftover insulin in these circumstances, very little extra sugar ends up stored as fat. In other words, all the sugars and the insulin get where they need to be and nothing gets left behind—or stored in the behind!

As we've discussed, some sugars, the refined carbs, aren't as good for you and aren't as easy for your body to manage. These sugars are like a bunch of tourists on vacation who are supposed to arrive at a theme park via tour bus. The problem is the tour bus didn't show up and now they're all trying to catch a ride in the taxis on the street. But because they weren't supposed to be riding in taxis in the first place, they are unprepared and don't have enough money for cab fare. This means that only a few of the tourists manage to get rides to the theme park and all the rest of the them are left standing at the curb.

Now think about our refined carbs. Like the tourists, the carbs (sugars) are supposed to get where they are supposed to go: in this case, by riding in the little insulin taxicabs. But because they aren't the right kind of sugars they get "left at the curb," without transportation to their designated destinations. Do you know what happens when refined sugars are left behind and standing at the curb? That's right, they get stored as fat. Even worse, when they end up stored as fat, the body doesn't have access to the energy or the hormones it needs to stay fit.

And that's not all. Do you know what else happens to the newly stored fat? Not much. In fact, it lounges around as long as you'll let it. And what makes matters even worse is that this fat is in all probability attached to a toxin you absorbed either from the environment or as the result of a by-product of one of the body's processes (as mentioned in the previous chapter). While most of us are concerned about the fat we can see on our outsides—the fat we so desperately want to get rid of—this fat is only a small part of the problem. Even more dangerous is the fat we can't see, the fat that is combined with toxins and that sticks around, because this is the fat that really causes major health issues. It's the fat you can't see in the mirror, the stuff that surrounds your vital organs, like the heart and liver, that is so dangerous. Plus, fat is one of the most difficult energy stores for the body to break down and use.

Fortunately, the body has a defense mechanism in place to help. This protective system is called muscle, and muscle is fat's biggest enemy. Why? Because it burns fat better than anything else. This means that the more muscle you have, the less fat you have. In simplistic terms: big abs, not big flabs.

How can you avoid this sugar problem and keep all your little insulin taxicabs running effectively and efficiently? Pay close attention to the amounts and types of sugars you eat and drink—and choose the best ones for good health. With the labels now required on all food products, it's easy to tell if what you're consuming is on the "unhealthy" list. If you start to feel sleepy before you finish reading the ingredient list on a product because it's so long, that's a good indication that it may not be all that good for you. One good rule of thumb is this: the shorter and simpler the list of ingredients and the easier they are to recognize, the easier it is for your body to utilize what's in the product effectively. If you take in high amounts of refined sugars and carbs into your body on a regular basis, you will only make your problem worse. In this case you'd be doing nothing more than "feeding the fat!"

In plain English, if a lot of what you are eating is the "junk" that you think tastes so good, you probably aren't eating enough of the stuff that's good for you. You can only be as healthy as each of your cells, and cells make up *everything* that you are: your organs, fluids, bone, skin, chemicals—everything. You have trillions of cells at any given time and your body continues to make new ones as old ones die and need to be replaced. If your cells aren't working correctly, nothing else will work as it should either.

...

So far I've tried to stick to my rule of providing basic information because generally I think that's all you really need to know and it's easier to remember that way. But the body is so far from simple that it's hard to imagine even a fraction of what really goes on inside of it. That's why for our purposes here I'm now going to share just one example of just how complex and complicated a cell actually is.

I've referred a couple of times to the "tiny bubbles" that make up things like hormones, nutrients, and insulin, right? And I've talked about how all of the tiny bubbles are made of cells, which are made of molecules. We've also discussed that we are made of cells and that different cells match different parts of the body.

Below is one example of what might be inside just one cell:

- 46 molecules of DNA (23 pairs of chromosomes)
- 10,000 to 100,000 different RNA molecules and proteins
- up to 100 million small molecules, such as glucose (sugar)
- 1 TRILLION molecules of water
- 2,500 mitochondria (powerhouses that generate most of the cell's energy supply)*

Does this description of a cell not blow you away with how sophisticated and complex our bodies are?

**The Molecules Within Us: Our Body in Health and Disease*, by Charles Pasternak, Perseus Publishing, 1998.

8

Hormone Imbalance & Nutritional Deficiencies

We have been talking about how important the type of foods we eat and nutrition are for our hormones and for good health. Now it's time to talk about the equally important subject of what happens when things get out of whack—in other words, when our hormones become imbalanced. Like I said before, when hormones are out of whack they don't work efficiently, and poorly functioning hormones can affect many key aspects of our overall ability to stay healthy.

Please bear with me as I use our cake example again. (I hope that all this talk about cake doesn't over-stimulate your taste buds, because while cake tastes good, it really isn't that good for you—whether you eat it a lot or eat a lot of it. Just for the record, though, let me say that I love cake. I just choose not to eat it very often and when I do eat it, I eat small pieces. That is, of course, unless it's white cake with real cream-cheese frosting or strawberry cake with real strawberries and cream-cheese frosting. Then even I have a hard time controlling myself.)

Anyway, back to our example. Think of your body as the cake that has to have very specific ingredients in exact amounts. Water is one of those ingredients because it is as important to your body as liquid of some kind is to a cake. Not enough water, or perhaps milk in the cake's case, and neither will be what it is supposed to be. To make a cake you also need all the other ingredients, like flour, baking powder, baking soda, salt, sugar, eggs, oil, flavorings, and so on. Leave an ingredient out or use the incorrect amount and your cake won't turn out the way you want it. It's the same with your body. Your body also needs to take in the right amounts of specific "ingredients." Just like the cake, if you don't get what you need or you don't get what you need in the correct amounts your body won't behave the way it's supposed to behave either.

We all know the first rule of survival is breathing. But after that, food comes in a pretty close second. Every living thing has to eat (to get its energy through some source) to survive. Therefore, what we eat should contain everything we need—that is, if we choose the right things to ingest. Vitamins and minerals are some of the substances we need that are in the foods we eat in differing amounts. Vitamins and minerals might be described as the building blocks for the body's countless processes. Because we rely on them so extensively, if we don't get enough of them we can pretty much be guaranteed that somewhere along the line our body will notice the lack. How will we know? Because it will start to function less and less well, breaking down in different ways to call our attention to the problem. In other words, poor eating habits bring about vitamin and mineral deficiencies that contribute to hormonal imbalances and poor health.

Vitamins and vitamin deficiencies

Below are a few examples of vitamin deficiencies and the results of those deficiencies. To determine if you are deficient in any of these vitamins, you will need to have a blood work panel performed with your health care provider.

The National Institutes of Health "Office of Dietary Supplement's Vitamin and Mineral Fact Sheets" can be good sources of information pertaining to sources of, and conditions related to, vitamins and minerals—or a lack thereof. These fact sheets were the resource for the following information.

Vitamin A

Vitamin A deficiency is seldom seen in the United States, but can lead to problems with the eyes, skin, teeth, and immune system. It can interfere with the development and maintenance of bone and with normal cell growth and development. Some of the foods with the highest vitamin A content are liver, sweet potato, carrot, mango, spinach, cantaloupe, dried apricot, milk, egg yolk, and mozzarella cheese.

One of the confusing things about vitamin A is that it occurs in two basic forms. Retinol is the preferred, active form of vitamin A, found in products that come from animals, such as liver, milk, cheese, cream, kidney, cod, halibut, and eggs. The other form of vitamin A, betacarotene, comes from the naturally dark colored dyes found in plants, such as carrot, pumpkin, sweet potato, winter squash, cantaloupe, pink grapefruit, apricot, broccoli, spinach, and most dark green, leafy vegetables. The brighter and deeper the color of a fruit or vegetable, the higher the levels of betacarotene. Betacarotene is a formidable antioxidant. *Antioxidants* are substances that protect cells against the effects of *free radicals*, molecules produced when the body breaks down food, or by environmental exposures to things like toxins, tobacco smoke, and radiation. Free radicals can damage cells and play a role in heart disease, cancer, and other diseases. We'll talk more about antioxidants and free radicals later in this book.

Vitamin A is one of the four vitamins that are referred to as "fat soluble." *Fat-soluble* means that the vitamins can dissolve in fat, a process that allows the body to store them for future use. That's why it's important to monitor not only the amount but also the form of vitamin A (and the other fat-soluble vitamins) we obtain through foods and supplementation. As with anything, too much of a good thing can be bad. In this case, too much of vitamin A in its "active" form, Retinol, can be toxic. The betacarotene form of vitamin A, however, is utilized by the body as it is needed and any excess is eliminated.

B complex (Thiamin (B1), Riboflavin (B2), Niacin (B3), Pyridoxine (B6), and Cobalamin (B12))

B complex is a vitamin with extensive benefits. While the list below is nowhere near complete, it should give you an idea of just how helpful this vitamin can be.

Healthy levels of B complex contribute to various bodily functions, such as: producing hormones; metabolizing fats/proteins; enhancing metal ability and IQ; protecting against cancer; balancing cholesterol, blood pressure, and blood sugar levels; protecting against arthritis, migraines, kidney stones, gallstones; avoiding/alleviating heart disease, cataracts, neurological disorders, depression, PMS, Alzheimer's and schizophrenia; stimulating sex drive; detoxifying pollutants, alcohol, narcotics, and lead; correcting metabolic imbalances caused by birth control ("the pill"); boosting athleticism; functioning as antioxidant; enhancing immune system function; and healing infections.

B complex vitamins are naturally found in animal products, including meat, poultry, fish, eggs, milk, and milk products. They can also be found in beans and some fruits and vegetables. To ensure you are getting adequate amounts of these crucial B vitamins, it's imperative to eat regular, healthy, well-balanced meals. Because B complex vitamins are essential *water-soluble* vitamins—that is, they cannot be made or stored in the body—we need to continually bring them in either through food or supplementation.

Vitamin D

Vitamin D is another fat-soluble vitamin whose deficiency can lead to a disruption in the way cells function. Given the trillions of cells that make up our hormones and bodies, we'd do well to remember to always get enough vitamin D. The greatest natural source of vitamin D is sunlight. As little as 5 to 10 minutes of a day of *direct* sunlight is all most of us need to produce enough vitamin D unless a disease or dysfunction interrupts its production. Interestingly, the color of our skin has an effect on vitamin D production. Someone who is considered fair-skinned may only need to spend about 45 minutes a week in the sun with her face and arms exposed to produce enough vitamin D. Someone who has dark skin, on the other hand, may need up to 3 hours of exposure to achieve the same benefit. The amount of sunlight that actually reaches the skin is also tempered by the clothes we wear and the application of sunscreen as well as amounts of cloud, shade, and smog cover in the environment. You might think that you could get your dose of vitamin D by sitting by a window with the sunlight coming through and hitting your skin, but this is not really true. The preferred way of getting vitamin D is to receive the sun's rays *directly onto your* skin as it allows for a much higher level of absorption.

It is estimated that as much as one third of the population lacks the ability to properly convert vitamin D from the sun (vitamin D2) into the usable form, vitamin D3. This means that even if you spend the suggested amount of time in the sun, you still may not be getting the benefits you require and why supplementing with the converted form of vitamin D3 is so crucial. Now aware of the benefits and the average individual's challenge to process vitamin D, some medical doctors have begun to prescribe supplements for their patients. My mother-in-law, for example, has been prescribed vitamin D supplements by her primary care physician. Although prices for these supplements are often high, you can find high-potency, high-purity vitamin D at very affordable prices without a prescription. (In our office, we personally recommend and carry two vitamin D products in their converted form. Neither contains soy and one of these products is organic.)

Once in the body, vitamin D is converted by the liver and kidneys into its usable form, called *calcitrol*, or D3. There are two dietary forms of vitamin D: *cholecalciferol* and *ergocalciferol.* These are found naturally in some foods and in fortified milk. The milk used to make yogurt and cheese is usually not vitamin D-fortified. Foods sources of vitamin D include cod liver oil; however, cod liver oil also often contains very high levels of vitamin A, which as mentioned can be toxic over time. Other good sources for vitamin D are fatty fish like tuna, salmon, sardines, mackerel, and herring, and eggs. Make sure your fish is "wild caught"—not "wild raised" or "caught fresh"—to help reduce toxin intake. Farm-raised fish should be avoided because it carries the highest risk for heavy metals, toxins, artificial colors, and additives.

I typically include vitamin D in my supplement regimentation, especially in the winter months, as I do EPA/DHA, or fish oil. And since vitamin D is fat-soluble, your body can store and then tap into any excess in your system if your levels start to run low. Vitamin D also affects how nerves and muscles work together, helps keep the immune system working properly, and has been shown to affect mood, sleep, and energy levels. Vitamin D deficiency has been shown to cause *rickets*, a childhood disease where bones are weak, causing them to bow or curve under pressure. In adults this syndrome is called *osteomalacia*, or "soft bones." As much as 85% of the population has been shown to be deficient in vitamin D, one of the highest rates of deficiency for all vitamins. If you have been tested and find you are deficient, drinking milk is not the answer for regaining proper levels. In fact you'd probably kill the cow trying to get enough. Generally speaking, good eating habits and the right vitamin D supplement are keys to maintaining proper levels.

Vitamin D has received its fair share of media attention because it is possible, though highly unlikely, to take too much. Too much vitamin D can result in potential negative side effects, including the possible interaction with some medications, tiredness, poor appetite, diarrhea, muscle problems, weight loss, frequent urination, constipation, excessive thirst, vomiting, bone pain, metallic taste in the mouth, itchy skin, and eye problems. It is therefore recommended that you take vitamin D under the supervision of a knowledgeable health care provider.

Remember, not all health care providers will have the relevant knowledge to help you make the right decisions in regards to vitamin supplementation. This is not an indication that you should forego supplementation altogether, however. Instead, find an informed individual and get the facts.

The growing awareness of how much our bodies rely on vitamin D has raised concern that the dietary recommended daily intake values (DRIs) put out by the USDA are woefully obsolete: 200 IU (International Units) a day for adults 19 to 50 years old; 400 IU for those 51 to 70; and 600 IU for those over 70. Experts now agree that the DRIs for vitamin D are way too low, particularly for people who don't get sufficient sun exposure. Some studies have shown that adults need anywhere from 3,000 to 5,000 IU per day, and that 10,000 IU can be metabolized without harmful side effects. But in order to be safe, limit your intakes and talk with your health care provider before you begin your supplementation regimen.

One of the most important things to remember is that you cannot get too much vitamin D if you're getting it from the sun or from the foods you eat. It's simply not possible. Monitoring vitamin D levels most effectively requires that blood tests be done on a regular basis. While it is recommended that the majority of us need to be supplementing with vitamin D, anyone with kidney disease, heart problems, or high phosphorous or calcium levels in the blood should not take vitamin D without discussing it first with a health care provider.

Vitamin E

Vitamin E is the third fat-soluble vitamin. (Vitamin K, necessary for the clotting of blood, is the fourth, but we won't be discussing it here.) The primary role of Vitamin E is as an antioxidant. Antioxidants are the nutrient substances that help us get rid of the free radicals mentioned briefly above. I will do my best to define what free radicals are and do first and then discuss why they are so important relative to vitamin E.

Free radicals

The body produces many, many different kinds of cells. Free radicals are cells that are naturally produced through normal functioning, but are dangerous to our health. They are created when the body breaks down the substances we eat, drink, and breathe and are absorbed through the skin or by environmental exposures to things like tobacco smoke, radiation, and chemicals. Regardless of what causes their production, however, they remain renegade cells in that they cause as much trouble and do as much harm as possible.

One important thing to know about cells is that they—along with every other part of the body—are controlled and enabled by electrical signals running through our bodies. If not for electricity our brain and heart would cease to work altogether. Furthermore, cells, along with everything else, are made up of atoms. Atoms are made up of protons, neutrons, and electrons. Protons have a positive charge, neutrons have a neutral charge, and electrons have a negative charge. When these charges are out of balance, atoms become either positively or negatively charged, just like a battery. The switch between one type of charge and the other allows electrons to flow from one atom to another. It is this flow of electrons, or negative charge, that we call electricity. When we talk about the nervous system sending "signals" to the brain, or the brain telling our hand to pick up a book, what we're talking about is electricity carrying messages between point A and point B.

The problem with free radicals is that their charges aren't balanced. It is this imbalance that makes them act, well, crazy. Imagine these cells rattling, shaking, and bouncing around all over the place in an attempt to "balance" themselves, while at the same time trying to steal the electricity they need from your healthy cells. Essentially, what happens is that during the process all this destructive activity damages the healthy cells. If the process doesn't kill the healthy cells outright, it can interfere with how the cells work too, something equally injurious. In essence, free radicals are like violent gang members who recruit new members every time they come in contact with another group, or "cell."

But now for the really scary part: once free radicals steal the energy from a normal cell, that cell ceases to perform the function it was meant to perform and may actually begin to harm your body instead. That cell then divides, as all cells do, and creates more damaged cells just like it. This opens the door for illness and diseases like cancer.

How does this relate to vitamin E? Vitamin E has antioxidant properties that fight the onset of free radicals. It is therefore a critical element for the body's ongoing health. Luckily, most of us probably get the vitamin E we need from the plant oils in the foods we eat and since vitamin E is fat-soluble our bodies do a pretty good job of storing it. Animal oils generally have no vitamin E; however, safflower, sunflower, soybean, corn, and wheat germ oils all contain the vitamin E your body needs to help it stay healthy. Asparagus, peanuts, green leafy vegetables, almonds, and sunflower seeds are all great sources of vitamin E as well.

Mineral deficiencies

Minerals have the same reciprocal relationship to hormone balance as vitamins. If you don't get enough of the right minerals and vitamins in the right amounts you may suffer the consequences of hormone imbalance, and hormone imbalance can rob your body of vital nutrients.

It might help to envision what minerals "look like" in the same way we pictured hormones, as tiny bubbles. Minerals play a vital role in the body's functions and processes and are important components in bone, muscle, skin, and other body tissues, and in fluids like blood and water.

You might tend to think of a mineral as something that comes from the ground or from rocks if you were to crush them. In that case you would be partially correct because the minerals that come from the things we eat, like vegetables and fruit, get their life-sustaining nutrients from the soil in which they grow. Fruits and vegetables are always good sources of minerals, but because they have a tendency to bind, or not release, the minerals from their tissues it can be difficult for the body to utilize them efficiently and effectively. Generally, meat and seafood are good sources because they have the highest concentrations of minerals. Furthermore, the minerals they contain are somewhat easier for the body to process and utilize.

Thirteen different minerals are necessary for the human body to get what it needs on a daily basis to ensure all the normal processes function as expected. These minerals are: calcium, magnesium, iodine, sodium, iron, potassium, zinc, copper, selenium, manganese, chloride, molybdenum, and phosphorous. Minerals are classified in two categories, either *major* or *trace*, depending on how much the body needs to function correctly. According to *Perspectives in Nutrition* (3rd edition) by Wardlaw and Insel, the 7 major minerals are (not in order of importance) sodium, potassium, chloride, calcium, phosphorus, magnesium, and sulfur. The body requires at least 100 milligrams (mg) of each of these minerals every day. 100 mg is the approximate equivalent of 1/50 of a teaspoon. It may be hard to comprehend that such small amounts are so vital for our functioning, but suffice it to say that even in these amounts minerals are invaluable to the body's overall health.

Trace minerals are different from major minerals in that they are required by the body in amounts *less than* 100 mg per day. The trace minerals are: iron, manganese, copper, fluoride, molybdenum, iodine, chromium, and selenium. Most of these minerals are required by the body in such miniscule amounts that it's almost impossible to imagine. In the end, what you need to know is that if you are eating *well-balanced* meals you are probably getting all the trace minerals you need.

What if you don't feel you're getting the right amount of minerals in your diet? Are you someone who doesn't like vegetables or meat? If that's the case, think about incorporating small amounts in your diet. It's true that certain minerals like potassium and magnesium are much more abundant in plants form—that is, in vegetables—than meat or seafood. But the key is to eat a *balanced* diet. The general consensus among scientists and one that is supported by most of the literature is that a well-balanced diet provides all the nutrition you need.

I personally find a flaw in this theory. First, there is an assumption that most of us eat a "well-balanced diet." This could not be further from the truth. In the U.S., for example, studies show that nutritious foods are sorely missing from the diet most of us eat day to day. Given the fact that in America over two thirds of our population is either overweight or obese, and the fact that we continue to see an increase in disease and dysfunction, we can assume only that the well-balanced diet is not the one on everyone's plate.

It is the fact that most of our diets are so *im*balanced that leads me to believe that most of us *do* need to supplement to help ensure our bodies get the nutrients we need. What supplements to take and for how long are considerations best made with the help of your health care provider. This is no easy task as many factors must be considered, but not meeting your body's needs or over-supplementing are both undesirable consequences that can leave you in a poor state of health.

Of course special circumstances exist where even the healthiest people may need to take an additional vitamin or mineral to meet a specific need. Women who are attempting to conceive or who are pregnant, for example, are often prescribed additional folic acid to support the proper development of the fetus and individuals with anemia (iron-poor blood) may need to supplement with additional iron. Again, I encourage you to enlist the help of a health care provider who can assist you in these matters.

As we said above, minerals are required in extremely small amounts. This begs the question: exactly how much of our overall body composition is made up of minerals? Authors James F. Balch, M.D. and Mark Stengler, N.D. of *Prescription for Natural Cures* tell us that minerals compose 4% of the body's weight. Sounds relatively insignificant, right? But consider the following: the body of a 125-pound individual should have approximately 5 pounds of minerals relative to total weight. The body of a 175-pound individual should have approximately 7 pounds of minerals. And 200 pounds of body weight should mean 8 pounds, and so on. If you weigh between 125 to 150 pounds, the weight of the minerals in your body should be equivalent to lugging around a backpack of 5 or 6 bags of flour or sugar all day.

Secondly, in terms of having a "balanced diet," even if you are attempting to eat in a way that supports good nutrition it can be challenging at best to meet your body's requirements based on the food we have available to us and consume in today's world. Instead, the overall poor quality of food products we ingest on a regular basis definitely supports our "garbage in, garbage out" paradigm. It's bad enough that the majority of us don't eat fruits or vegetables daily (or even regularly) and that even those who do generally eat one serving a day compared to the minimum 5 or 6 we should be eating. But add to that reality the fact that our fruits and vegetables are grown in soil whose mineral content has become so depleted of nutrients—so lacking in critical vitamins and minerals—that we usually can't get what we need from them no matter how much we might eat! With that said, since research shows that the nutritional value is higher in organic produce than conventionally grown fruit and vegetables found in most supermarkets, we would all be best served by eating organically grown foods whenever possible.

Eating organically

Here is a good example of how eating organically can change your life. You may find the information eye-opening; I see it as further evidence that what we eat can have devastating effects on our health. The study cited below was published in the *Journal of Applied Nutri-*

tion (45:35–39) and was titled "Organic foods versus supermarket foods: Element levels." Researchers compared the amounts of both "healthful" and "toxic" minerals in organically and conventionally grown foods and found the following.

Healthy minerals

The following minerals have been found to exist in higher quantities in organically grown foods, as indicated by the percentages.

- boron: 70% higher in organically grown foods
- calcium: 63% higher
- chromium: 78% higher
- cobalt: same in both groups foods
- copper: 48% higher
- iodine: 73% higher
- iron: 59% higher
- lithium: 118% higher
- molybdenum: 68% higher
- nickel: 66% higher
- phosphorous: 91% higher
- potassium: 125% higher
- rubidium: 28% higher in conventionally grown foods (not a desirable mineral)
- selenium: 390% higher
- silicon: 86% higher
- sodium: 159% higher
- strontium: 133% higher
- sulfur: 20% higher
- vanadium: 8% higher
- zinc: 60% higher

Toxic minerals

The following minerals have been found to exist in higher quantities in non-organically, or conventionally, grown foods, as indicated by the percentages.

- aluminum: 40% higher in conventionally grown foods
- cadmium: 5% higher
- lead: 29% higher
- mercury: 25% higher

Now let's take a brief look at 4 of the 13 of major minerals, namely calcium, zinc, magnesium, and potassium.

Calcium

Calcium is the most abundant mineral in the human body, constituting approximately 40% of all the minerals stored. Calcium has several important functions. For example, nearly 99% of the body's total calcium is stored in the bones and teeth, where it functions to keep them strong and hard. The remaining store of calcium can be found throughout the body in blood, muscle, and in the fluid between cells. Calcium supports other processes as well, such as muscle contraction, blood-vessel contraction and expansion, the secretion of hormones and enzymes, and the sending of messages through the nervous system. A constant level of calcium in the body's fluid and tissues is necessary for these vital processes to keep functioning efficiently.

Although dairy products are the main source of calcium in diets across the United States, other foods also contribute to our overall calcium intake. For individuals who do not enjoy dairy products, who are lactose intolerant (cannot completely digest milk sugar, or lactose, and experience symptoms like bloating and diarrhea), or who are vegan (don't eat animal products) and avoid or have completely eliminated dairy products from their diets, meeting calcium needs through alternative sources is critical.

Chinese cabbage, kale, and broccoli are excellent sources of calcium. Although most grains are not high in calcium (unless fortified), because they are ordinarily consumed frequently, they do contribute a small amount of calcium to most diets. Additionally, there are several calcium-fortified food sources presently available on the market, including fruit juices, fruit drinks, tofu (soybean) products, and cereals.

As the *2000 Dietary Guidelines for Americans* states, "Different foods contain different nutrients and other healthful substances. The following are strategies and tips to help you meet your calcium needs each day:

- Use low-fat or fat-free milk instead of water in recipes, such as pancakes, mashed potatoes, pudding and instant, hot breakfast cereals.
- Blend a fruit smoothie made with low-fat or fat-free yogurt for a great breakfast.
- Sprinkle grated low-fat or fat-free cheese on salad, soup, or pasta.
- Choose low-fat or fat-free milk instead of carbonated soft drinks.
- Serve raw fruits and vegetables with a low-fat or fat-free yogurt-based dip.
- Create a vegetable stir-fry and toss in diced 'calcium-set' tofu (a concentrated source of calcium).
- Enjoy a parfait with fruit and low-fat or fat-free yogurt.
- Complement your diet with calcium-fortified foods, such as certain cereals, orange juice, and soy beverages."

One important fact is that estrogen plays a critical role in the absorption of calcium. How well calcium is absorbed in the small intestine depends greatly on having a sufficient amount of the active form of the vitamin D hormone, calcitriol, present. Estrogen is essential for the synthesis (the combining of different parts to make a whole) of all the things necessary to form calcitriol and to the absorption of the calcium. Calcium is most readily available to the body for absorption in a more acidic environment. When an environment has a pH level of 6 or lower, it is considered more acidic than alkaline. (The scale of relative pH values goes from 1 to 14, with 0 being the most acidic.) Most calcium absorption occurs in the upper part of the small intestine, also known as the *duodenum*, where the pH level is typically around 6.

Zinc

Zinc is an essential mineral that supports the function of at least 300 enzymes within the body. Again, "essential" vitamins and minerals are those that the body cannot make own and therefore must be taken in through foods and/or supplementation. Remember, enzymes are molecules that increase the rate of chemical reactions inside cells. Using our Los Angeles street analogy, enzymes are the traffic cops, directing traffic in different directions at different speeds so that all involved get where they need to go as soon as possible. Zinc is critical in allowing the enzymes to do the job they need to do.

Zinc appears in a wide variety of foods. Oysters contain more zinc per serving than any other food, but red meat and poultry provide the majority of zinc in the American diet. Other good food sources include beans, nuts, certain types of seafood, such as crab and lobster, whole grains, fortified breakfast cereals, and dairy products, although some of these foods are difficult to absorb due to the presence of *phytates*. Phytates are phosphorus compounds, found primarily in cereal grains, legumes, and nuts, that bind with minerals like zinc, iron, and calcium. Because phytates interfere with the absorption of minerals in the body and the availability of zinc from grains and plant foods is lower than that from animal foods, we need to get most of our zinc from other sources.

Zinc is one of the principle protectors of the immune system and hence is a major fighter of disease. Think of zinc as a general in the armed forces battling against all the bad stuff like cold viruses and bacteria, while also supporting all the other "troops" of the immune system. In the event you suffer an injury like a cut or a scrape, zinc can help your immune system fight the infection and support faster healing of the wound. Zinc also acts as an anti-inflammatory, both in and outside the body.

Zinc has also been found to contribute dramatically to normal growth processes, whereas an insufficient level of zinc in the body can reveal itself in symptoms such as a decreased sense of smell, taste, or appetite, hair loss, diarrhea, and an acne-like rash. Zinc has been found to impede macular degeneration (an eye disorder that damages the center of the retina, called the *macula*, and makes it difficult to see fine detail) and assist in maintaining vision, help in the treatment of acne and in the prevention of hair loss, and maintain the ability to taste and smell. Zinc is also required for the body's production of numerous hormones and is necessary for proper reproductive development and fertility.

Magnesium

Magnesium is the fourth most abundant mineral in the body and is equally essential for good health. Approximately 50 to 60% of total body magnesium is found in bone. The other half is found predominantly inside the cells of tissues and organs and circulating in the blood.

Magnesium, a requirement for more than 300 biochemical reactions in the body, helps maintain normal muscle and nerve function, keeps the heart's rhythm steady, supports a healthy immune system, and keeps bones strong. Magnesium also helps regulate blood-sugar levels, promotes normal blood pressure, and is known to be involved in energy metabolism and building protein. Currently, scientists are looking at the role of magnesium in preventing and managing a number of disorders, such as hypertension, cardiovascular disease, and diabetes. Magnesium deficiency can be revealed in symptoms of an irregular heartbeat, weakness, disorientation, and muscle pain. In some instances seizures have also been known to occur.

What foods are good sources of magnesium? All green vegetables, because they have high levels of chlorophyll (which contains magnesium) and gives them their green color. Some legumes (beans and peas), nuts and seeds, and whole, unrefined grains are also good sources of magnesium.

Refined grains are generally low in magnesium (and most other vitamins and minerals). As the process of refining and processing white flour removes the healthy parts of the flour, such as the magnesium-rich germ and bran, it's always preferable to eat breads made from whole-grain wheat flour because it has many more nutrients. Additionally, most processed breads are made with "bleached" flour. The term *bleached* means exactly that: the wheat has been bleached in the same way you might bleach your white clothes to clean them. Since labels on bleach bottles plainly worn us of the dangers not only of skin contact with bleach but of ingesting this powerful substance, I feel distinctly unmotivated to willingly put it in my body in the form of bread or any other "bleached" food product.

Tap water is another potential source of magnesium (and other minerals), but amounts vary according to the water supply. Water that naturally contains a higher mineral content is described as "hard," and contains more magnesium than "soft" water. Hard water often has enough magnesium in it that it can be considered a food source in its own right, but tap water generally also contains chlorine, a substance added to help kill dangerous bacteria. Since chlorine in sufficient quantities becomes toxic, the drawbacks of drinking chlorinated water may outweigh the benefits of a higher mineral content. The best thing to do before you decide to use your tap water as your source of magnesium—or for anything else—is to verify just how "good" it is. Local water departments have testing facilities where you can have water samples tested for contaminants to determine levels of things like fecal matter (human waste), prescription drug levels, heavy metals, and so on. We personally no longer use our tap water for cooking or drinking and are installing a main-line filter for the entire house to ensure our water is pure for bathing as well.

You may be familiar with the fact that magnesium can be helpful in bone health, too (according to the National Institutes of Health). Most of my patients who are concerned about the health of their bones are looking for or are already taking some type of supplement that contains magnesium as well as calcium. While it's true that these are both very important minerals for bone growth, there is another, called MCHC, or microcrystalline calcium hydroxyapatite compound, that is at least as critical. Let's refer to my favorite analogy of baking a cake once again to make our point. MCHC is to bone what flour or sweetener is to cake; in other words, a key component. I therefore recommend it be incorporated into any supplementation program for this purpose.

Magnesium also helps maintain healthy muscle and can be used to treat neuromuscular disorders (those that affect the nerves that control voluntary muscles), to lessen the symptoms of premenstrual syndrome (PMS), and to help fight depression. Healthy levels of magnesium benefit the entire system by helping to protect against cardiovascular disease, treat high blood pressure and nervous disorders, prevent kidney and gall stones, and control diarrhea, vomiting, and indigestion (which, if excessive or chronic, can eventually lead to magnesium deficiency). Magnesium is also important for energy production and breaking down glucose, or sugars, in the body.

The National Institutes of Health also states that even though dietary surveys have suggested that many Americans do not consume recommended amounts of magnesium, symptoms of magnesium deficiency are rarely seen in the United States. Concern remains, however, about the fact that there is a prevalence of suboptimal magnesium stores in our bodies because less-than-required levels of magnesium indicate that we do not have the amount we need to effectively protect against disorders like cardiovascular disease and immune dysfunction.

Because magnesium is absorbed in the intestines and then transported through the blood to cells and tissues, the health of the digestive system and the kidneys is significantly influenced by the status of our magnesium levels. Only about one third to one half of the magnesium we take in through dietary sources is actually absorbed into the body. Furthermore, gastrointestinal disorders that impair absorption, such as Crohn's disease, can also limit the body's ability to absorb magnesium by depleting the body's stores. In extreme cases, this may result in magnesium deficiency. The excessive loss of magnesium through the passing of urine, sometimes a side effect of taking certain medications and in cases of poorly controlled diabetes or alcohol abuse, can also result in magnesium deficiency. Conversely, a healthy set of kidneys can limit the urinary excretion of magnesium and can effectively compensate for a low dietary intake.

Potassium

Potassium is often called the "banana mineral" because it's long been a common recommendation to eat a banana if experiencing cramps or muscle aches. Potassium has a direct relation to sodium (salt) levels in the body as they work together to help maintain the body's fluid balance. Sodium is found primarily outside the cells, while potassium is found almost exclusively inside the cells. In addition to balancing fluids, the two help move nerve impulses in the form of "messages" or sensations from the brain to the nerve ending and back again.

Because the body absorbs about 90% of the potassium contained in whatever we eat, it seldom needs to be supplemented. For this reason, however, you will want to pay attention to the potassium levels that occur naturally in what you eat as it is rarely added to foods that are processed. Great natural sources for potassium are green, leafy vegetables, tomatoes, oranges, broccoli, peaches, avocados, potatoes, squash, legumes/beans, bananas, whole grains, and meats. Luckily for many Americans, potatoes retain potassium even in the form of French fries (although the quality of the potatoes and the oils used will effect—or detract from—their overall health benefit) and potassium even exists in coffee, tea, and milk.

Because potassium plays such a critical role in regulating nerve impulses, fluid balance, and muscle activity it follows that it is also extremely important for women as it pertains to hormonal imbalance and its side effects, such as cramps, bloating, dehydration, nausea, and fatigue—just to restate a few. For most people potassium insufficiency is not a concern. If you take diuretics, however, drugs usually prescribed to help control high blood pressure and tend to increase urination, it would be prudent to take note of your potassium intake and levels. Either way, a severe enough imbalance in potassium levels can result in outcomes like kidney failure. Potassium levels have been seen to drop to dangerously low levels with diuretic use, but also with eating disorders, such as anorexia and bulimia, where the body does not get or maintain the potassium it needs. Even athletes, who consistently perspire more than most of us, and people who live in extremely hot climates have to be careful not to suffer from the effects of potassium deficiency.

9

To Supplement or Not To Supplement

Now that we've discussed how critical vitamins, minerals, and all nutrients are to our hormone health and our overall health (which of course are really one in the same), the question becomes: should you supplement or not?

The use of dietary supplements continues to be a source of widespread discussion, especially within the medical community. It seems many doctors refuse to discuss their use with their patients and some go so far as to advise against taking them.

From a primary care physician's viewpoint, it's hard to argue the point. Unless they have spent time researching the benefits of supplementation, at best most M.D.s may have had one or two nutrition classes somewhere towards the beginning of their educational process. This means that things like vitamins, minerals, essential fatty acids/fish oils, and the best foods to eat and why are generally not the main focus of their practice. These physicians are usually far more knowledgeable in diagnosing illness and prescribing medication, since these are the areas in which they have the most training and experience.

If you are someone who has found yourself confused and perhaps frustrated at the reluctance of your doctor to address the topic of supplementation—or to address it positively—I understand. Especially in light of the fact that the *Journal of the American Medical Association*, the "bible" of the medical establishment, shared its view on supplements over eight years ago. In this landmark article published in June 2002, the *Journal of The American Medical Association* (*JAMA*), the medical community's most prestigious research publication, announced that all adults would do well to take vitamin supplements to help prevent chronic diseases. "Suboptimal folic acid levels, along with suboptimal levels of vitamins B6 and B12, are a risk factor for cardiovascular disease, neural tube defects, and colon and breast cancer; low levels of vitamin D contribute to osteopenia and fractures; and low levels of the antioxidant vitamins (vitamins A, E, and C) may increase risk for several chronic diseases. Most people do not consume an optimal amount of all vitamins by diet alone. It appears prudent for all adults to take vitamin supplements," the article's authors, Robert H. Fletcher, M.D., M.Sc, and Kathleen M. Fairfield, M.D., Ph.D., stated.

Just a few years ago you would have had to look long and hard to find a primary care physician, let alone a specialist, recommending or prescribing a supplement. Those that did were in the vast minority. The great news is that things have started to change.

As we advance in knowledge it is becoming more common to find the greater medical community recommending supplements to its patients, especially those with heart and cardiovascular conditions, intestinal issues, such as constipation, diarrhea, irritable bowel, Crohn's disease, leaky gut, and sometimes for those taking antibiotics. For heart and cardiovascular issues, fish oil (EPA/DHA) is now commonly prescribed and probiotics are recommended on limited occasions for intestinal issues and for antibiotic therapy.

Vitamin choice

How should adults who haven't been taking vitamins go about choosing the right ones? The Dietary Supplement Information Bureau (DSIB), a nonprofit information resource created specifically to provide consumers with scientifically accurate up-to-date information, offers some practical advice. According to Dr. Jeffrey Blumberg, a member of the DSIB Scientific Advisory Board and a nutrition scientist who is an authority on disease prevention through vitamin supplementation, here are some guidelines for choosing vitamins:

Take multivitamins, as recommended in the *JAMA* study, if you are an adult. Choose a "multivitamin" that contains minerals as well as vitamins.

Read the ingredients panel on your supplement carefully. Your goal is to come as close as possible to the RDA (Required Daily Allowance), the minimum daily requirement of each vitamin and mineral your body needs.

Remember to take your vitamins every day, preferably with meals. Taking them only occasionally or seasonally is not as effective.

Check the label for ALL required vitamins and minerals. Additional supplements may be required to achieve the minimum daily requirement of certain ones (calcium, for example) beyond the amount contained in any multivitamin. (cont.)

Check the expiration date on the bottle. All reliable companies date stamp their products.

Consider formulations made specifically for your age group and life stage. There are multivitamins designed for children, adults, seniors, and for pregnant women.

Select a brand name you trust. Health care professionals can provide advice on brands.

In our clinic we have recommended and urged patients to use supplementation when necessary for years. Unfortunately, the nutritional values of our current food supply, even of organic foods, are well below what they were 20 years ago and substantially lower than they were 50 years ago. Amazingly, it has been estimated that our current food products may lose as much as 90% of their nutritional value by the time we eat them. This is in large part due to the fact that our soil has lost its rich mineral content through overuse and lack of replenishment. Plus, as mentioned earlier, we now have a tendency to overcook just about everything we eat, a process that further robs our foods of the nutrients we need. The microwave, while convenient, may be the worst offender of all.

In a recent webinar, Joe Buishas, CCN, LDN, of the Healing Oasis Wellness Center in Wisconsin, shared insight on this topic. "In 1914 an apple contained almost half the minimum daily requirement of iron, but today you would have to eat 26 apples to get the same amount. Iron is not the only nutrient depleted. In 80 years apples have declined in the following minerals: the amount of calcium in apples has dropped 48%, phosphorous is down 84%, iron 96%, and magnesium, the famous heart nutrient, has dropped 82%. The amount of calcium has declined 81% in cabbage, 92% in lettuce, 56% in spinach, and 48% in apples. During the same time period, magnesium levels have dropped by 77% in cabbage, 91% in lettuce, and 35% in spinach. Iron levels dropped from 60% to 99% in the same vegetables."

My wife Kylee and I have been taking supplements for a long time. We personally take fish oil and vitamin D on a consistent basis, plus probiotics to help maintain a healthy intestinal tract and immune system. I believe these are essential for the body to help it perform as it was intended. We also undertake a detoxification program at least a couple of times a year for the same reason.

Where should you get your supplements? Because no supplement is yet under the auspices of the FDA, consumers are at the mercy of the companies that make them. Given the recent dramatic increase in the interest in health, weight loss, and wellness, the supplement industry has seen a boom in business. Whenever this happens in any industry there are companies who get involved who have no real expertise in the field. The same is true with supplements. You can pretty much buy them anywhere you shop, including your corner convenience store.

I have a rule I follow when it comes to my supplements: I don't buy my nutritional supplements anywhere I can buy a candy bar, toilet paper, or have my oil changed. But that still doesn't necessarily make buying a good-quality supplement simple. Since the FDA or any other governing body is not involved, companies are on the honor code to ensure that the ingredients they say are in a product actually are in it, in the amounts they claim, and of quality grade.

A common question I get from patients is, "How do I know if I'm getting a good supplement and not wasting my money?" That, of course, is the million-dollar question or, in the case of the supplement industry, the billion-dollar question. Given how complex and daunting a task it is to find high-quality supplements, I can only encourage you to leave it to those who know the most about it. Naturally, that raises the next big question: who exactly would that be?

This question can also be very difficult to answer with any certainty. That's why I have spent years researching supplements and their constituents. As a result of my research, I only deal with supplement companies that sell to licensed physicians; in other words, I do not buy from retail companies that sell to retail stores over the counter.

First of all, I buy only from companies that can provide me with proof of the quality and concentration of their products. They can do this because they actually invest part of their profits back into research and development with the goal of ensuring their ongoing commitment to quality and consistency—the quality and consistency we all deserve. None of us should expect anything less from the makers of our supplements.

Secondly, I buy my supplements only from specific companies that have their products tested by an independent third party. This third party performs an assay, or analysis, to determine the characteristics and components of the supplements on a regular basis, a process that helps make sure that all of the claims made on the company's product labels are accurate.

Lastly, the companies where we get our supplements produce them in a facility whose operating methods and procedures are certified. This also helps ensure we are getting what is referred to in the supplement business as "pharmaceutical grade" products. This is as important for supplements as it is for prescription drugs. For example, for any given medical condition a doctor prescribes a certain medication in a specific dosage for the patient to take for a certain period of time. This is done based on research undertaken by the pharmaceutical company that has shown that, within certain parameters, a specific drug in a specific amount over a given period of time will likely produce a specific outcome. In the simplest terms, this means if you take your medicine as prescribed by the doctor, you should see prescribed results. The same is true for supplements as well.

There are a number of other considerations for dealing with the companies we do, but these are the most important. The reason I have spent so much time researching and finding the right suppliers is because it is so important for my health, my family's health, and the health of my patients and their families. I would never ask one of my patients to take a product that I would not take or recommend for my family.

...

Our discussion about nutrients, food, fat, and their relationship to hormones will now lead us to a deeper discussion about the different types, or groups, of hormones. This information should provide a solid foundation to better understand what hormones really are and how they affect you.

Review

Before we move on, let's do a quick review of what we've covered so far:

1. Your brain and your nervous and endocrine systems work with and control your hormones.
2. Hormones affect how you feel physically and mentally and how healthy you are.
3. Hormones are made of nutrients.
4. Nutrients come from what you eat.
5. What you eat, the amount you eat, and your body's ability to absorb and break it down are primary factors in how much fat your body produces and your overall health.
6. The type of carbohydrates you eat affect your insulin "taxicabs."
7. Fat can affect all body processes, including your ability to produce the right amount of hormones and whether or not you are able to produce healthy hormones.
8. The right fats in the correct amounts are required for optimal health.
9. Excess fats, sugars, and carbohydrates are stored in the body.
10. Most often, fats are stored attached to some type of toxin.
11. Vitamin and mineral deficiencies can be associated with hormone imbalances.

PART TWO

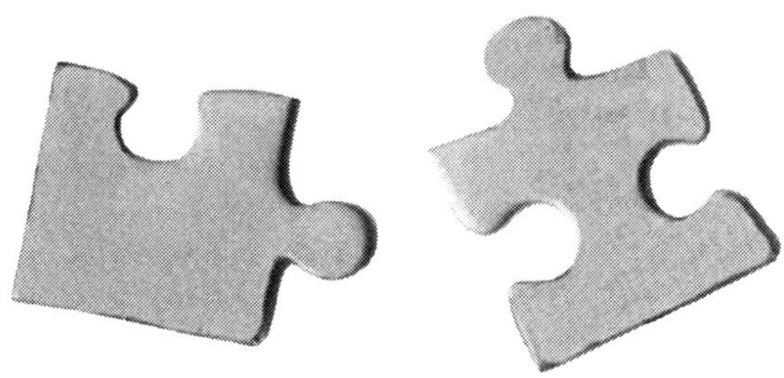

THE WORLD OF HORMONES

10

YOU'RE ALL MESSED UP & WHO'S TO BLAME

X*eno-*, *eco-*, *synthetic*, *bioidentical*, and *natural*: all are types of hormones. But don't let the unfamiliar words scare you; I promised to keep it simple and I will. You will be surprised how easy it is to understand the cool stuff going on inside your body and controlling your every function even as you are reading this book.

In an *ideal* environment, the body produces all the hormones it needs naturally in exactly the right amounts and at exactly the right time and has all the parts it needs and none of the parts it doesn't. That means that everything has been put inside you for a reason, whether you or modern medicine knows what that reason is.

For example, just a few years ago scientists found a new muscle that attaches the skull to the covering of the spinal cord. Research has only recently revealed that this newly discovered muscle may be a cause of headaches and migraines when it isn't functioning properly. It's hard to believe that after all the thousands of years that scientists have been studying the human body and with all the medical advancements we've made in this last century alone, this little muscle went undetected, isn't it? But this is just one of many new discoveries that will continue to be made. That's why any "expert" on the human body and how it functions will tell you that as much as we continue to learn there is much, much more to know.

Which brings me to a very important point. Just because you don't know what some part of the body does or what it is for doesn't mean you don't need it. For some reason or another, whether we know why or not, every part we have has a purpose. If these parts do not work correctly, we can be assured that at some point or another, in some way or another, we will see the effect in the form of some symptom, disease, or dysfunction. Again, in an ideal environment, we would all be in "perfect health"—though we as humans really have no real way of knowing what that means. Because in the real world—where we all live—none of our bodies is in perfect health. In fact, I would venture to say that most of them are in a state a lot less than perfect.

Finger pointing

If you would like to know who or what to blame for why your body is in the condition it's in, you might want to start pointing fingers because there are probably very few things that *haven't* affected you in some way, whether it's the water you drink, the food you eat, or your entry into the world at the moment of childbirth. The most important thing is to realize that when you point one finger there are always three fingers pointing back at you. What do I mean by that? That as much as we'd like to place the blame for our unfortunate circumstances (and whatever they are, we all have them) somewhere else, if we are honest we need to admit that we ourselves are as much to blame—probably several times over.

It seems as though humans tend to forget a critical element of living life: that we are accountable to and for ourselves. We are responsible for our actions, reactions, thoughts, words, and emotions and how they impact each one of us individually, our environment, and the lives of those around us.

You may want to point a finger of blame at the fast food industry—and justifiably so—for degrading the health of the general public. But let's face it. No one forces us to eat fast food. We all have a choice. Your kids (if you have them), on the other hand, may not. If the only places you take them to eat are places that serve food of poor quality with poor to no nutritional value, that's where they'll eat. (That's Finger Number 1.) Second, fast food restaurants cannot affect your health or your waistline if you don't eat their food. (Finger Number 2.) And, finally, if you eat fast food on a regular basis, you are only supporting the corporations that provide it. (Finger Number 3.) I actually believe "colluding" might be a more appropriate word in this case because you personally are choosing to support the industry's decisions and standards, or lack of them. And don't forget, when I say "fast food" I also mean a great deal of the food sold in the grocery stores that, nutritionally speaking, isn't worth the packing it comes in.

But perhaps it's not your eating habits but your stress that you blame for your current situation. After all, stress is an underlying component in virtually every disease or dysfunction of the body and more and more studies are being done that prove this to be true. Maybe it's your family that causes you stress. We can all relate to that, right? Or if you are in school, you may want to point the finger at a particularly tough teacher or trouble with another student. If you're working, maybe it's your boss or a coworker who aggravates you. Maybe it's too much homework or too big a workload being thrown your way. Maybe you have a difficult time getting along with people, or keeping to a schedule, or maybe you're just plain stressed out because of all life's clutter. Whatever the reason, one thing is for sure: it is the rare individual who would not say that his or her life is stressful to one degree or another.

Life's clutter

"Life's clutter" is all the stuff that complicates your daily life. Generally it makes you feel as if your head is spinning. When you're overwhelmed with this kind of clutter, you can't seem to get anything done; you're generally tired and not all that happy, at least for the most part. Life's clutter is all the stuff from home, work, school, social groups, family, and the environment that piles up and leaves you feeling that it's hard to move in the direction you are meant to go. It keeps you from living the life you want to be, and are meant to be, living.

My point here is that we can point a finger wherever we want in this situation, but the three pointing back at us remind us of who controls our lives and the amount of clutter in it: we do. If we think we don't, we have allowed ourselves to become so overwhelmed by our own clutter that we can't see the difference.

For the purposes of this book, however, we need to look at some of the things that might be making it harder for us to do what is in our best interest and how to change them. And since these things are probably at least partially affecting our health and hormones, it's really not altogether wrong to send a little of the blame in their direction. First and foremost on the problem front are environmental toxins.

A dangerous world

We've touched on toxins already to some degree, but will now discuss them more in depth. Remember, a toxin by definition is a poison. And, simply put, poison is poisonous. There's no way of getting around it. Poisons can never, ever be good for you. There's no in between. Though the effects of a poison may depend on how much we get of it, there is not one poison that is less than 100% bad.

The truth is that everything we eat, drink, breath, and absorb through our skin affects us to a point. We don't have to be consciously aware of how the substance enters our body or how much of it is entering our body for it to produce whatever effect it will produce either. And it's just possible that if we knew how many toxic substances had the potential to affect us every single day most of us would be afraid to leave our beds in the morning.

Luckily for us, what we do know gives us the option of doing something about it. Sometimes it takes only a second to clue us in to the fact that something's not right. For example, most of us know right away when we taste something rotten, eat something that doesn't agree with us, or breathe in the scent of something that doesn't smell the way it should. When that happens, we can simply throw it away or decide to stay away from that substance altogether now and in the future. In the moment, though, our bodies may experience any of a number of possible reactions, anything from nausea to vomiting to a burning sensation to hives on the skin—all signs that we have come in contact with some sort of toxin. The reason the body reacts is to let you know; in other words, to protect you. In actuality, millions, if not trillions, of these actions and reactions occur both in and on the body all the time, but most take place at the cellular level where we have no conscious knowledge of them. That's because our bodies are brilliantly created to process, break down, and discharge the toxic junk they come in contact with before it does too much real harm. And to some degree that's exactly what they do.

How much can our bodies handle before they can't keep up anymore? Good question.

It is no coincidence that as the modernized world continues to experience phenomenal advances in every aspect of our lives it is also seeing some disturbing side effects of that same progress: the quality of our foods has diminished; disease rates, in many cases, have increased dramatically; and the environment is suffering worldwide. Technological advancements purport enhanced lifestyles, but one could certainly argue whether that perspective is really a valid one. One of the laws of physics is that for every action there is an equal and opposite reaction, and I would have to say this is a case in point.

But while the situation may seem futile and hope like a stab in the dark, I believe things *can* get better. We *can* make a difference. We just need to know how.

It all starts with our health. The better we feel, the better those around us will feel, and so on, where the pattern goes into a kind of automatic regeneration. We've all been around people who feel so good that they make us feel good too; it happens all the time. What we all need to do is take notice of how it feels, focus on how it works, and take up the cause ourselves. When we feel good, we do good things, and those good things can—and often do—have a global impact.

And now, more on toxins and their relationship to hormones.

11

DANGER! DANGER!
(THE DANGERS OF ENVIRONMENTAL HORMONES)

Many of the toxins we encounter are called *xeno-hormones* or, more commonly, *eco-hornmones*. "Xeno" is from the Greek, meaning "strange," "foreign," or "different." "Eco" also comes from the Greek, from *oikos*, the word for "house." Most of us recognize *ecology* as the branch of biology concerned with the relationship of organisms to one another and to their physical surroundings. In today's world, "eco" is a common prefix to many words; it has generally taken on the meaning of anything to do with nature and is often used synonymously with "green."

In a medical context, xeno-hormones (or eco-hormones) are also called *endocrine disruptors* and are a large class of exogenous compounds: compounds that are produced outside the body. The primary problem with endocrine disruptors is that they damage developing tissues in the endocrine system. This includes the thyroid and pituitary glands, the adrenal glands, the testicles and ovaries, and the pancreas (which produces insulin). Damaged tissue can ultimately lead to major health problems, dysfunction, disease, and even death. In other words, although we associate "eco" with anything ecologically "friendly," in this case it is nothing of the sort. Rather, these hormones are environmental hazards created from our modern, "technologically advanced" world of plastics and pesticides.

Persistent organic pollutants (POPs)

POPS, or persistent organic pollutants, are also xeno-hormones. These compounds are difficult, if not impossible, for the environment to dissolve. Because they are so durable, they are capable of hitching rides and traveling great distances via rain, wind, storms, animals, and humans. This process has a significant impact on both human health and the health of the environment.

Many pollutants travel such long distances that they have been found in Antarctica, thousands of miles from any source that could have produced them. This is just a single example of how seemingly small things, such as one factory's production of PVC pipe, or another's production of toothbrushes, rubber ducks, or widgets, can significantly impact the entire planet.

One example of a persistent organic pollutant that is part of this poisonous cycle is the mercury that continues to pollute our rivers, lakes, streams, oceans—and bodies. First, microorganisms and the smaller "fish foods" absorb the mercury from the water and other food substances. Then, once the mercury-polluted organism/toxin has been absorbed by the fish, it begins to grow in concentration. As bigger fish eat the smaller fish, the level of toxicity magnifies and then magnifies again, and again (et cetera), until the toxic fish is eventually eaten by humans. This process of the food chain is known as *bioaccumulation* and *magnification.* Unfortunately, even if the days of industrial and commercial "dumping" of mercury, other heavy metals, and toxins into our streams, rivers, and lakes were to become a thing of the past, these substances would not disappear. Though they do degrade somewhat over time, they never *biodegrade*, which means they remain virtually unchanged in the environment (water or earth), with the exception of size, forever. And as we know, any health threat to the fish we eat ultimately becomes a health threat to us as well.

I'm not saying don't eat fish. Because fish provide essential fatty acids (EPAs and DHAs) required by our bodies' cells to maintain good health, and because the body can't make essential fatty acids on its own, fish are considered a vital and necessary part of most good eating plans. Some types of fish, however, are less likely to carry contaminants than others. The worst culprits are often the denser, more oily fish like swordfish, tuna, or mahi-mahi. "Wild-caught" fish is less likely to have the contaminants and chemicals often found in farm-raised fish. Don't be confused or misled by the term "wild raised," however. Wild-raised fish can pose some of the same threats as farm-raised fish, and is not at all the same as the "wild-caught" variety.

What are some of the negative and potentially harmful aspects of farm-raised seafood? Many species of farm-raised fish are raised in horribly overcrowded pens with little room to swim freely as they would in the wild. As with any species, restriction of movement can lead to poor overall health. Just think of the unhappy gorillas in their cages in the zoo. Furthermore, overcrowding means the fish virtually swim in and ingest their own excrement. This high-bacterial environment then requires the fish be treated with antibiotics to kill the bacteria. As we've already discussed, drugs and toxins are stored in the body. This is true for fish as well. That means that when fish are given food that is polluted with toxic endocrine-disrupting chemicals (like antibiotics), it ends up stored in their meatiest parts. The humans that eat these fish are then on the receiving end of those same toxic chemicals. In farm-raised salmon, for example, it is a common practice to feed the fish dye so that their meat will appear pink, as it would in their naturally occurring wild counterparts. If the meat of this salmon were not dyed pink, it would have an unhealthy gray pallor—something most of us would likely turn our noses up at.

When you consider we aren't the only animals that eat fish, it's easy to appreciate the greater environmental impact this process of bioaccumulation has as well. Birds, bears, otters, beavers, snakes, raccoons, skunks, and possums are just some of the creatures that eat fish as part of their regular diets. When these animals are consumed by other animals, the problem is only exacerbated, right on up the food chain. It's impossible to know the true scope of this poisoning magnification and how it will truly affect our world in the future.

In May 1995, the United Nations Environment Program (UNEP) Governing Council began investigating persistent organic pollutants. It found that many POPs are currently still in use in pesticides, in industrial products (such as solvents and polyvinyl chloride (PVC), and in pharmaceuticals. Given how many prescriptions Americans use, the potential level of human exposure to POPs relative to pharmaceuticals alone is staggering.

POPs and pharmaceuticals

In order to get a clear idea of how significantly pharmaceuticals affect our world, we need to look at the big picture. A 2007 report entitled "IMS Health Reports Global Prescription Sales Grew 6.4 Percent in 2007, to $712 Billion" from IMS Health, the world's leading provider of market intelligence to the pharmaceutical and health care industries, stated that the "total global prescription market [was] estimated at $712 billion based on sales, an increase of $178 billion over the past five years." The report also revealed that America was still the largest market of pharmaceuticals with total sales of $286.5 billion, a figure almost double that of any other country. To put this in perspective, Europe's top five markets—France, Germany, the United Kingdom, Italy and Spain combined—reported sales of $140 billion, followed by Japan at $65.2 billion.

We aren't just *spending* too much on prescription drugs either; the fact is that we may be using much more than we need. A major effect of being part of a culture that relies so heavily on pharmaceuticals containing POPs is that the drugs we take are likely disrupting the functioning and health of the endocrine systems of the general population.

But prescription drugs are just one source of these toxic pollutants. Our day-to-day lives are filled with examples of xeno- and eco-hormones that we come in contact with. We will list a few of the major sources here.

Pesticides

Most pesticides, from the ones we use in our yards and gardens to the types used in commercial applications are squarely on this list. Sometimes it is easy to forget that every single non-organic fruit and vegetable you buy in the store or eat in a restaurant has been grown to maturity using pesticides and chemicals. And, while it is true that using pesticides helps keep all the little critters away and makes the foods we eat look appealing, their use also has a significant downside as well.

Plastics

Next on our list are plastics. One of our greatest exposures to persistent organic pollutants/endocrine disruptors is through plastics of all kinds. It may surprise you to learn, since we continue to produce them and use them to such a great extent, that plastics are inherently toxic. For example, there has been some recent negative publicity around microwaving food in plastic containers due to the resultant exposure to toxins released in the heating process. Studies have confirmed that heating foods in plastic causes the leaching of the toxins into the food itself—whether it's leftovers for supper or your baby's milk. Even the storage of foods in plastic containers, though convenient, has been found to increase our susceptibility to plastic toxicity.

A good example of a toxin that acts as a hormone disruptor is the chemical Bisphenol A, or BPA. BPA, a long-used additive to some plastics, has been widely publicized as highly toxic to all living species. Many companies have agreed to stop using BPA in their products and many stores, such as Walmart, have stopped selling products that contain BPA due to its potential dangers. It's good to know that any product that contains BPA must reveal that fact by having the number "7" on the bottom inside a small triangle of arrows, the recycling symbol now found on many products. But don't be fooled. BPA is only one of the toxic elements that contribute to the chemical composition of plastic. So, just because a plastic product does not contain BPA, it still contains other POPs and endocrine disruptors that may be just as toxic. What does this mean? While you may be protecting yourself against one poison, you are still at risk for contact with numerous others.

The list goes on. Your exposure to potentially harmful pollutants in the form of plastic also includes the siding on and the wiring in many houses and the plumbing through which both your drinking water and bathing water run.

Bisphenol A: Recycling Symbol 7.

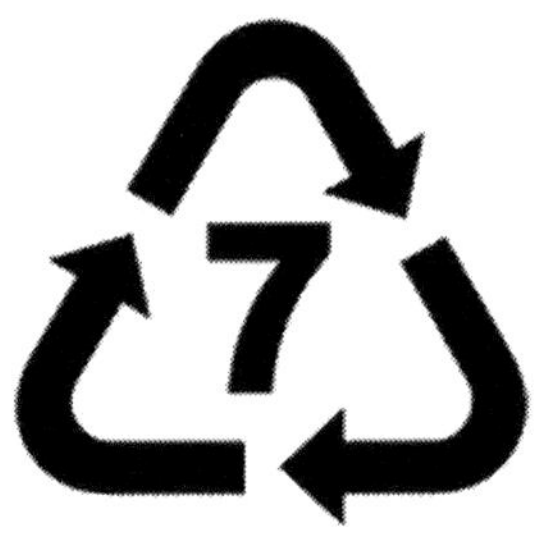

Plastics and their derivatives are found in flooring, roofing, carpeting, upholstery, insulation, your clothing, and the cosmetics and body products you wear and that are absorbed into your skin throughout the day. And this is just a small sampling of the plastics that bombard you while you are "safe" at home.

All of your furniture, whether it's made from wood, cloth, or leather, is loaded with potentially harmful substances. And if the chemicals used to make, preserve, or color the furniture aren't enough, almost every potentially flammable item in our homes today has been treated with a fire retardant, a substance that easily makes the list of probable troublemakers for the body. And if you think that none of this really affects you or the environment, a quick look on the Internet will show you that flame-retardant chemicals are already showing up in the fish in our oceans. Ignoring the impact technology is having—and could have in the future—on everything we use, from foods to plastics, doesn't change the facts. Sadly, it won't change the potential outcomes either.

We also need to add electronics to our list, as they are a source of persistent organic pollutants as well. It wasn't long ago that a typical American home had perhaps one radio, one phone, and a record player. Over the last 30 or so years that scenario has changed dramatically to the point where electronics are everywhere. We have a phone in every room so no one misses a call—or has to travel very far to answer it. This is in addition to all the cell phones we now can't live without for every member of the family, particularly if there are preteens and teens around. Then there are gaming boxes, DVD players, stereo components, remote controls for every gadget, electronic juicers, coffee makers, bread makers, toasters, alarm clocks.... The list never ends.

Gone are the days of one television set per household. It seems that every household has to have at least two televisions, often many more; I personally know people who have them in every bedroom, living room, dining room, and kitchen—along with complementary DVD players. And if you're thinking, "Well, at least they're not putting one in the bathroom," think again. I have a very good friend who did (although it's actually really cool, hidden behind a mirror).

If you are one of the lucky ones who has somehow managed to avoid most of this electronic overload, the time you are not wasting using them may leave you plenty of time to clean house. But if you just heaved a big sigh of relief, you might want to reconsider because in all probability the cleaners you're using are also brimming with toxic, endocrine-disrupting, persistent organic pollutants that can enter your system much more easily and much faster than those from all the electronics put together. So much for the big sighs, right? Every sigh may be shortening your life.

Friendly cleaning products

On the topic of cleaning products, however, you're in luck. More and more options are currently available in terms of products that are not only more friendly for the environment but also more friendly to you and your pets. Until relatively recently it was somewhat difficult to find organic food, let alone organic household products. But that has changed, where now you can get pretty much anything and everything you need for the house without sacrificing your health. We made the choice some time ago to go "green" and organic as much as possible, not only with the food that we eat but the household products we use as well. Again, this is very much a personal choice that each person and family has to make on his, her, or its own. Personally, we feel the small difference in price is well worth the benefits to our health and the environment. Be aware, though, that many "natural" cleaning products are no safer than their alternatives. As with food products, "natural" does not automatically mean organic or "safe," so *read the labels.*

Earth-friendly organic and natural cleaners work just as well as the other stuff, too. They are less toxic, if not completely non-toxic, and have none of the residual chemical odors. And I can assure you I have not noticed any crazy things growing in our house or strange buildups of grit or grime with their use. Our clothes are clean and no one has referred to us as "the stinky family" (at least not so we could hear). What I *have* noticed is that when we clean with these products, the air smells clean and fresh and not as if a fleet of tanker trucks headed to the toxic-waste dump just drove through our house.

When we repainted a couple of rooms recently, we chose a paint that doesn't contain VOCs, the volatile organic compounds contained in most paints. These toxic substances are responsible for that "new paint smell" and continue to be released for years after the smell goes away. It may be hard to believe, but the EPA reports that indoor air is three times more polluted than the air outdoors, and that the VOCs in paint and varnishes are some of the leading causes of indoor pollution.

Other toxic pollutants

If all this information about endocrine-disrupting, persistent organic pollutants turning your house into a death trap is alarming, maybe you should go out and sit in the fresh air by the pool, which is full of clean, clear water. Right?

Wrong. First of all, the air is anything but fresh unless you live on a mountaintop or a beach. Even then it's questionable, but probably better than the house smog you were inhaling. And the pool water is only clear and "clean" due to the chemicals added to it on a regular basis, such as chlorine, which is definitely not good for anybody. (Just think about the bleach.) The swimsuit you wear with that great print of bright colors is another concern, as it is probably made with a fabric that contains toxins, fabric that inevitably gets its color from dyes, that, unless they are all-natural, are also made from toxins. And your towel, spread out on the pool-side chair (likely made of 100% plastic and/or vinyl as well), probably contains POPs in its fiber and dyes, too.

Next, you put on your sunglasses. By now you won't be surprised to hear that most sunglasses are made of plastics or plastic derivatives. If you proceed to coat yourself in sunscreen to avoid damage to your skin, your dismay may ratchet up a notch when you hear that many of the ingredients in your sunscreen are on the list of toxic endocrine disruptors. Last but not least, let's swim over to your float and the pool toys that are all, you guessed it, made from plastics containing a variety of persistent organic pollutants.

There are a few natural sources of persistent organic pollutants, but most are created in the industrial and manufacturing processes. And the majority of the more than 2,000 chemicals that flood the market every year do not go through even the simplest tests to determine toxicity. This is according to the Natural Resources Defense Council.

Paranoid yet? Me, too. I'd tell you to take a deep breath and relax, but knowing what I just told you about the air both inside and outside, unless you have access to pure oxygen, I wouldn't advise it.

But panicking isn't the answer either. There are things you can do, so read on.

12

Toxins and Their Horrible Effects

After hearing about how dangerous and prolific persistent organic pollutants are, your next question should be, "How exactly might these endocrine-disrupting, toxic hormones be affecting me?" As we've already discussed, exposure to persistent organic pollutants takes place through things you knowingly—or unknowingly—put in or on your body, environmental exposure, or accidents. These exposures have many potential effects—the worst one, obviously, being death. Short of death, however, exposure can cause serious illness, including disruption of the endocrine, reproductive, and immune systems, neurobehavioral disorders (disorders that have to do with the way the brain affects emotion, behavior, and learning), and cancers of all kinds. I believe exposure to POPs is a major factor in the increasing numbers of allergies, asthma, abnormal monthly periods, difficulties in pregnancy, chronic fatigue, fibromyalgia, and generalized aches and pains our society is experiencing. I also believe it's entirely possible that toxic exposure could be contributing to conditions such as depression, ADHD, autism, and other brain and nerve disorders.

A study published in the journal *Diabetes Care* in 2006 (29:1638–1644) supports suppositions like these. Researchers in this case found a link between blood serum levels of POPs and diabetes, where individuals with elevated levels of persistent organic pollutants (DDT, dioxins, PCBs, and chlordane, among others) in their bodies were found to be up to 38 times more likely to be insulin-resistant than individuals with low levels of these pollutants. This makes sense when we are reminded of just how important our little insulin "taxicabs" are to our health.

Numerous studies continue to reveal that we all are walking chemical cocktails of contaminants. According to the Centers for Disease Control (CDC, www.cdc.gov) *2005 National Report on Human Exposure to Environmental Chemicals*, Americans retain dozens of chemicals from pesticides, consumer products, and cigarette smoke in their blood and tissue. In its third report, when the CDC checked 2,400 people for 148 chemicals it found more than 90% had a mix of pesticides in their systems. And although almost everyone is contaminated to some degree with phthalates, substances added to plastics to increase their flexibility, transparency, durability, and longevity, children appear to carry a bigger load of phthalates and of pesticides than adults.

Phthalates

And speaking of phthalates.... Phthalates are chemicals used in a large variety of products, including the coatings of pharmaceutical pills, and in industrial and manufacturing settings to control qualities like consistency and gelling properties. Phthalates act as lubricants and binders to emulsify and suspend various agents. Everyday uses of phthalates include adhesive and glue products, agricultural applications, building materials, personal-care products, detergents and soaps, paints, printing inks and coatings, food products, pesticides, and textiles. It's bad enough that there are pesticides on and in the fruits and vegetables that end up inside us, but what about all the chemicals inside our food products, soaps, lotions, and makeup?

The CDC's *Third National Report* list adds a number of common sources of phthalates to my list, including soft, plastic fishing lures, nail polish, caulk, and toys made of so-called "jelly rubber." Phthalates are found in shower curtains, perfumes, modern electronics, and medical applications like catheters. The most widely used phthalate is found in PVC (polyvinyl chloride), which is used for the majority of all plumbing materials due to its low cost.

Since 2004, it is estimated that manufacturers have produced about 363,000 metric tons (800 million pounds) of phthalates. That equates roughly to a little over 2.5 pounds of phthalate produced per American, per year. Would anyone like my share? No, I thought not.

It is more than a little scary that this toxic chemical is used in everyday products like toys and makeup. And it's a lot scary when we begin to question whether our body has the ability to effectively process and rid itself of all the poisonous substances that infiltrate it. Our bodies are amazingly resilient and powerful, it's true, and capable of detoxifying a lot of what we ingest, apply, or otherwise encounter. But with the amounts bombarding our bodies day in and day out, every single day of our lives and with the apparent increase in diseases and dysfunctions we are seeing worldwide, we can only assume that these poisons are taking a serious toll on our health.

Detoxification

With all the stuff—both good and bad—that goes into the body, there has to be some way of removing what becomes waste. For this purpose, the body has a detoxification system in place. Detoxification, the removal of toxic substances from the body, is the body's way of attempting to return to a natural state of balance, or homeostasis, and is part of the body's natural process. The body's primary method for detoxifying occurs through the liver, but detoxification also takes place in the lungs, skin, blood, kidneys, and other organs.

Think of all the diseases and conditions that can affect any or all of those organs. Given the toxins with which we continually come in contact, it's hard to imagine how our bodies can detoxify to the degree we need them to in order for us to stay healthy. The frightening thing is, it's quite possible they cannot.

While it's true that we have many choices about what we bring into our lives, sometimes we have no choice. Some contaminants are passed from our parents to us during conception, for example, and some are present when we enter the "sterilized" world of the hospital. Our tiny little systems not only go through the unbelievable shock of the birth process, but contact with hundreds of toxins in every plastic, rubber, metal, and fabric it meets, right down to the soft blanket that wraps it. Unless you were born under very unusual circumstances, I'll bet you dollars to doughnuts not one of these products was organic or chemical-free.

And so our little toxic journey begins. Knowing what you know now about all the sources of the toxins in your life, you can fill in your own list. Sadly, your first ingested dose of chemical contaminants may have come directly from the chemical-riddled baby formula you were fed immediately after birth. It's incredible, I know, but some brands of baby formula have been found to contain a chemical that is also used in jet fuel. It's hard to imagine why on earth a chemical used in the fuel that powers jets would be part of the formula for fuel that powers babies, isn't it? And we know that baby formula includes preservatives and additives, comes in plastic bottles, is drunk from rubber nipples, and is often microwaved to boot. Does anyone really need more proof that nourishment the way Mother Nature intended—through breast-feeding—is the best, most complete, whole-food source for an infant whenever possible? I understand breast-feeding is not always possible for a variety of reasons, but this is an example of how "advances" may not always be the best thing for our health and wellbeing in the long run.

For many of us, our artificial formula joined forces with our most treasured friend, the pacifier, early on in our development. Unfortunately, this toxic little twin of the rubber nipple—and call it what you will (I have heard plenty of descriptors over the years, including binky, plug, and passy)—is basically nothing more than a hunk of chewy chemicals. I guess what I'm saying is that one would have to question how good it is for a baby or a small child's system to be chewing on a chemical cocktail all day long. I know it's just one little thing and I know I've said it before. But little things add up, and sometimes they add up to big things that can be very, very dangerous.

Think about it for a minute. If you believe small things like pacifiers can't possibly do any harm because they're so small, try to imagine how big they'd be if they were made for adults. (Of course, giant pacifiers could be the answer to a lot of tense people's problems; on the other hand, the nipple of an adult pacifier would have to be about as big around as a rolling pin, not to mention that the mouth guard would really get in the way of our mobile phone usage.) But, just to make the point, keep that analogy in mind and consider the potential for ingesting toxins if we all went around sucking on a piece of plastic all day the way some infants and toddlers suck on theirs. (Of course now that I think about it, a lot of us are, given our addiction to plastic water bottles.)

I know a lot of you are saying to yourselves, "Right, you try to deal with a screaming kid without a pacifier!" (and that's deleting any expletives you might use). I understand your concerns, and I'm not telling you to use pacifiers or not. In fact, my daughter Alex used one because at the time I didn't know any better. I'm just saying pacifiers are just one more thing that we give to our children that might not be that good for them. Unfortunately, to this point there really aren't many options. (Although I can't let the opportunity go by without saying that people got along just fine without man-made pacifiers for thousands of years, relying on the ones Mother Nature gave to all women). One bit of good news is that my wife and I recently saw a pacifier made only from "natural rubber." This product's label listed no additional ingredients. Not that "pure rubber" is a great health benefit to the body either, but I think it's at least another option and one more little thing that you can do to help reduce your baby's toxic overload.

A study published in the February 2008 edition of *Pediatrics* suggests that some baby lotions, baby powders, and baby shampoos are exposing babies to phthalates as well. "We found that reported use of baby lotion, baby shampoo, and baby powder was associated with increased concentrations of monethyl phthalate (MEP), monomethyl phthalate (MMP), and monoisobutyl phthalate (MIBP) in infant urine," said the study's researcher, Dr. Sheela Sathyanarayana. This association was strongest in young infants under 8 months old, "who may be more vulnerable to developmental and reproductive toxicity of phthalates," the report noted. Dr. Sathyanarayana further pointed out that at present, U.S. manufacturers are not required to list phthalate contents on the labels of packaged products, something that makes it hard for parents to make informed decisions. "If parents want to decrease exposures for their children," she said, "they can try to use lotions, shampoo, and baby powder sparingly, unless otherwise indicated for a medical reason." Perhaps we should instead buy products that cleanse our babies' tender bodies without the use of toxic substances?

As you think about the list of chemicals and toxins that you have come in contact with throughout infancy, adolescence, and now adulthood, don't forget all the settings where they're found: in hospitals, at home, at school, in the playground, in the car—not to mention in the air you take into your lungs.

And don't forget that to get where you are now you've had to eat and drink and breathe for as long as you've been alive. It's discouraging to think about all the things we've put into our bodies that were—and conceivably are—riddled with preservatives, additives, and chemicals, presumably to make them taste better, smell better, look better, and last longer than they might otherwise. Did you know that many of the chemicals found in the foods you eat have been banned in many other parts of the world? It makes you wonder why we need them if other countries think they're so bad that they're worthy of banning. Why do we need yellow, red, and blue dyes and other dangerous chemicals in anything that we eat? I'll tell you why. Marketing. Appearance and taste sells, and boy, have we been sold.

When I was young I don't think things were quite so bad. The fast food revolution had just begun, as had the discovery and manufacture of many of the chemicals we use today. That's why I have to believe it is many times worse for kids now who are being brought up in a world where their food options tend to be between McDonald's and Taco Bell and their option to breathe clean air has all but disappeared. Remember, things add up over time. Where are *your* totals? Where will they be a year from now if you don't make any changes?

Generally, young kids don't get to make many of the decisions affecting their health, wellbeing, and life; their parents make those decisions for them. If you're a parent, knowing what you do now (which barely scratches the surface of what there is to know and is important to know), are you comfortable bearing the burden for "voluntarily" exposing your children to so much? Some things are out of your control, but many decisions are not. Do it for them. When you do, you may be encouraging them to take a different path. This can help them grow up making more educated decisions that could positively affect them, their own families, and their world.

13

MARGARINE & MCDONALD'S

If you have any doubt about what chemicals and preservatives do to the foods we eat—and hence our bodies—just do what I call The McDonald's Test. If you're like me, you'll be amazed, shocked, and disgusted all at the same time. To be fair, you can probably use any fast-food chain for your test, but I first saw this done with a McDonald's cheeseburger Happy Meal, and that's the meal on which I subsequently performed the test myself. You may have seen a similar experiment in a video version online recently, too.

Here's what you do. Go to McDonald's and buy the cheeseburger Happy Meal or any comparable meal. Take it home and put it in a place where no animals, rodents, kids, husbands, or anything or anyone can get to it. DO NOT REFRIGERATE IT! Take it out of the bag and its packaging and let it sit untouched right where it is.

You're probably thinking what I thought: "Ew, gross! How long before I won't be able to stand the smell of rotting food?" And you'll probably be just as astounded as I was because the answer is "NEVER." That's right. You will *never* smell the rancid odor of rotting meat or cheese and you will *never* smell the sickly odor from decrepit potatoes, or French fries. Why? Because they don't decay. These "foods," and I use the term very loosely, are virtually indestructible! They don't break down, they don't rot, and they certainly don't biodegrade! The last time I performed this experiment in our clinic, my specimen sat for just over eight months before I tossed it out of boredom. When I did, it hit the bottom of the wastebasket with a resounding *thunk*, just like a rock. And that's what we're putting in our bodies!

Furthermore, even more amazingly, even after eight months, there was literally virtually no change in the appearance of this "meal." The bun appeared as "fresh" as the day it had been purchased, but it was so hard I could thump it with my finger and not make a dent. In my first tests, I made sure to separate the top bun from the meat and cheese so I could track the progress of the decay that I was certain would occur. While the meat did eventually darken somewhat and may have shrunk slightly in size, those were the only changes I could see with the naked eye. The cheese remained relatively the same as well; again, it may have decreased slightly in size and may have been a little darker shade of orange-yellow, but there was no other evidence of change. I repeat. Nada. No change.

The French fries were also still pretty much picture perfect after the eight months of my experiment. Every single fry was the same perfect golden brown, and still appeared to "glisten"—believe it or not—with that famous sunshiny glow. If I had placed this meal side by side with another bought the day I ended my test, I honestly don't think anyone would have been able to tell the difference between the two. Terrifying, isn't it? Several of my patients didn't believe me when I told them about my results, so they tried it on their own. They were as flabbergasted as I was.

But if you don't want to take the time to do this experiment, try the margarine test instead; it's faster.

We all know that especially in the summer non-refrigerated dairy and vegetable-based products spoil relatively quickly. Leave a gallon of milk, a package of cheese, or even tomatoes or bananas on the counter (or, worse, in the sun) and see what happens. The flies that swarm around the food and the accompanying stench are fast and unpleasant reminders that it's been left out too long. *This is normal.*

Here's what you do to perform the margarine test. Take your tub of margarine, remove the lid, and set it outside when the temperature gets up into the 70s, 80s, or 90s. Position it so that it can receive direct sunlight for at least part of the day in order to speed up the experiment. One of the first things you will notice is that in most cases the margarine will melt; that is, it will change from its solid form to a liquid. What you probably *won't* see are flies.

I've performed this experiment myself and was shocked when I never saw even one fly come anywhere near the once rich, creamy, golden spread that people slather all over just about everything they eat. That means it didn't rot and it didn't degrade. It simply changed form by collapsing in on itself.

What I think we have to ask ourselves is this: if, even in its non-refrigerated, "degraded" condition, the flies literally won't touch it, why would we want to eat it when it's still "fresh"—whatever that means. The reason the flies aren't the slightest bit interested is because this "food product" doesn't exude a scent. It doesn't decay because it isn't real. It just sits on the table—*or in our stomachs and intestines and livers*—and sits and sits and sits. The reason? You guessed it: preservatives, chemicals, and processing.

So what's the point of these unscientific experiments? To me it's a no-brainer. If a food product contains enough preservatives and additives to keep it from breaking down even after eight months on a shelf or after setting it in the hot sun for an extended period of time, how much "nutrition" could it possibly have when we eat it? Could this be why so many people in our wealthy country are considered "malnourished?" What possible effects could these "foods" be having on our bodies? Frankly, after seeing this type of test with my own eyes I'd have to ask, *Who would want to find out?*

It's uncomfortable, and I'm not proud of it, but I'll confess that I was as big a fan of margarine and McDonald's as anyone before I performed my little tests. I didn't have one particular Mickey-D favorite, but I did have an affinity for the Filet-O-Fish meal, followed by the plain old cheeseburger, and then the Big Mac. Rounding out my favs was the Quarter Pounder with cheese, no onion. Man, did I miss them all when I stopped getting my fix on a regular basis. I wasn't sure exactly what they did to get them to taste the way they did consistently and to make me want to go back over and over again for more, but it worked. I was a repeat offender.

But please note the use of the word "was."

What I have since learned is that there is actually a scientific answer to explain exactly what kept me—and continues to keep millions—going back for more on a daily basis. A significant part of this answer comes in the form of one substance, called monosodium glutamate, or MSG.

MSG

I know you've all heard of it. MSG was first reported to have been used in the form of seaweed by the Japanese as a flavor enhancer. It was when other countries began to explore the reasons that seaweed added flavor to other foods that the discovery of its chemical counterpart, MSG, came about. MSG apparently made its debut in America sometime in the 1940s and by the 1960s its use had become widespread. Most of us know it in the context of Americanized Chinese food but MSG became a household name a long time prior to that in the form of a product you may also recognize: Accent. I remember that all the years I was growing up on our farm, Mom kept a bottle of Accent in the cabinet as a staple. I continue to tell myself that Mom's amazing home-cooking was a result of the farm-raised ingredients and her "special touch," and not due to the chemical enhancement of the Accent.

Today MSG is consistently found in a huge percentage of the foods available to us, the ones that line our shelves and we eat in restaurants, especially fast food restaurants. For many years MSG has been reported by the food industry to be a "safe" additive, and that its primary function is to "increase flavor as much as 80 to 100%." Unfortunately, this is only the tip of the addiction iceberg. First, this statement about increasing flavor begs the question: if the food is so good, why do we need to enhance its flavor by 80 to 100%? Good food should likely stand on its own, don't you think? Secondly, increasing the flavor of anything to such a great degree would seem to automatically make it much more appealing. So much so that one might almost say that it now becomes *addictive.*

And that's exactly the point.

It turns out that, according to many scientific studies, MSG is literally an addictive substance. This means that MSG does more than affect the taste buds and sensory centers of the brain; it affects all the other chemical reactions of the body as well.

What is this "miracle" additive? Monosodium glutamate is a by-product of glutamic acid, also known as glutamate, an amino acid. Yes, these are the same amino acids we talked about earlier, the ones that combine to form proteins and are found in plants and animals, including humans. When we speak of the glutamate in humans we refer to it as glutamic acid, L-glutamate, or L-glutamic acid. Glutamate in this form is 100% pure—in other words, free of impurities—a critical element of its ability to function appropriately in the body. MSG, however, is the "impure" form of glutamate (impure up to approximately 3%), so-called because it is processed, manufactured, and sometimes fermented in chemical laboratories. It is this impure, chemically induced form that is added to our processed and prepared foods that is cause for our concern. Then why do so many of our food products contain it? It's really quite simple: the more we eat of the food, the more we want. The more we want, the more we buy—whether it's French fries, macaroni and cheese, or tacos.

You may be curious as to why such a small amount of impurity—only about 3%—causes the body to react so negatively over time. The reason is that glutamate/glutamic acid is a *neurotransmitter*, one of the body's messengers that communicate information to and from the brain and all other parts of the body and make sure that those messages are correct. As we know, hormones like estrogen and progesterone are all neurotransmitters. Now imagine all these messages that are being carried by all these neurotransmitters traveling through the same nervous system. Because the nervous system does not differentiate between natural or manufactured neurotransmitters, the body's pathways are traveled by both alike. Since MSG is an *excitotoxin*, an agent that binds to nerve cell receptors, stimulates cells, and damages or causes their death, we should all stop to think long and hard about whether we want that particular substance running around our system with our other neurotransmitters, potentially wreaking havoc as it goes.

Because it is the MSG you ingest through the foods you eat that is of the greatest concern, you can avoid it by eating foods that have nothing added, such as raw fruits and vegetables and foods that are prepared without MSG. Sometimes you may not know if there is MSG in the food you're eating. In this case, feel free to ask. Restaurants should answer your question honestly and most times you can request they prepare your order without adding MSG.

Why don't you hear more about monosodium glutamate? Because MSG sales are a mainstay in a billion-dollar food industry. Furthermore, if we all woke up tomorrow without it most of the fast-food industry would collapse because its food would lose all the "flavor" it needs to sell it. In effect, it would taste horrible, seeing as most of it is made of substances that aren't real, at least by my standards.

Most of us want to steer clear of things that we know are damaging to our bodies and this includes substances that have the potential to kill our cells. Remember, you are only as healthy as each of your cells. If the food you're eating is killing off your cells, the bottom line is that it is killing you, too.

I know this information probably won't put a dent in the annual sales of margarine, McDonald's, or the Chinese food industry (not that all Chinese restaurants use MSG). But that's not why I'm sharing it with you now. The reason I've offered these examples is so that if you care to repeat these tests and see the results for yourself you can, or if you want to do a little more investigating on your own about MSG and how it affects you, you now know where to look. Then it's up to you to make your own deductions and decisions. Information in and of itself is useless until it's understood and applied. In this case, your life just may depend on it.

PART THREE

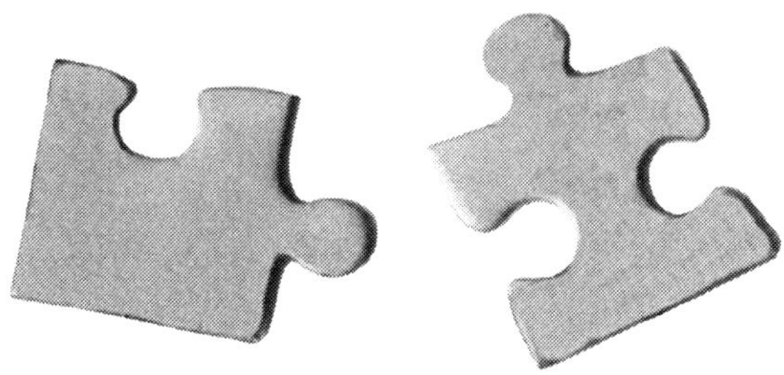

The Truth About Hormones

14

Detoxifying: Getting It All Out

By now you have figured out there is no escaping the onslaught of poisons we face from the environment. Even if you lived in a bubble, it would inevitably be made from plastic, so your attempt to escape the problem would literally put you right in the middle of it. Given that there is no possible way to avoid all the things that are bad, if not potentially lethal, to your system, what can you do?

First, you can limit your exposure. Eating organic foods, drinking purified water, and using organic products (makeup, cleaning supplies, and so on) puts a big dent in the status quo. Second, while there has been and probably always will be a debate on the "need" to detoxify or cleanse our bodily systems, I am a firm believer in the process. Our family goes through a major detoxification at least twice a year. There are literally hundreds of detoxification, or cleansing, programs and methods on the market. The programs we use are research-based and available only through licensed health care providers, such as chiropractors and medical doctors. While detox programs can have great benefits, they can still be dangerous if not performed correctly, so please work with a professional if you choose to undertake one. For more information on this topic, please log on to our website, www.hormonebasics.com.

Lastly, if you do decide to detoxify on your own (again, something I don't personally recommend), please do extensive research and choose the products you use wisely. One critical element of any cleanse is knowing any potential dangerous and/or negative side effects associated with that particular product. As with dietary/nutritional supplements, cleansing and detox programs are not yet fully regulated by the FDA, so there is no real accountability of the companies marketing those programs. Provided they don't do more harm than good, many of the products may result in your paying to virtually flush them down the toilet because they pass right through you without any real benefit—that is, unless a change in urine color or odor can be considered a benefit.

The products acquired through a trusted health care provider are usually of higher quality and of pharmaceutical grade to help ensure that you get what you pay for, that it will work as it was formulated to work, and that it has been produced to reduce any negative risks relative to the products and procedures involved.

15

NATURAL VERSUS SYNTHETIC HORMONES

Now that you know more about eco-/xeno-environmental hormones and toxins, it's time to learn more about the natural hormones you produce inside your own body, as well as the synthetic or bioidentical hormones that may be prescribed for you by your doctor.

Natural hormones are made *in* your body, *by* your body. *Synthetic hormones* are prescribed by your doctor and are chemically produced in a factory and patented for profit. They are similar to your own natural hormones, but they are not exactly the same. *Bioidentical hormones*, on the other hand, are manufactured in the lab to have the same molecular structure as the hormones made by your own body. Most bioidentical hormones are derived from soybean or wild yam plants. Because they are not considered "synthetic" there is some consensus that bioidentical hormones will not have the same side effects. Bioidentical hormones in any form should be prescribed by your medical doctor and obtained from a compounding pharmacy. We will discuss each of these types of hormones below.

Natural hormones

Although all of the more than 50 hormones in the body vary in terms of what they do, how they are intended to work, and by virtue of the different steps or "pathways" that are required to create them, they all have one thing in common: they are all derived from cholesterol. The following diagram shows the specific path that must be followed to produce the specific hormones we are talking about in this book: progesterone, the estrogens, DHEA, testosterone and cortisol.

Hormone Creation Pathways.

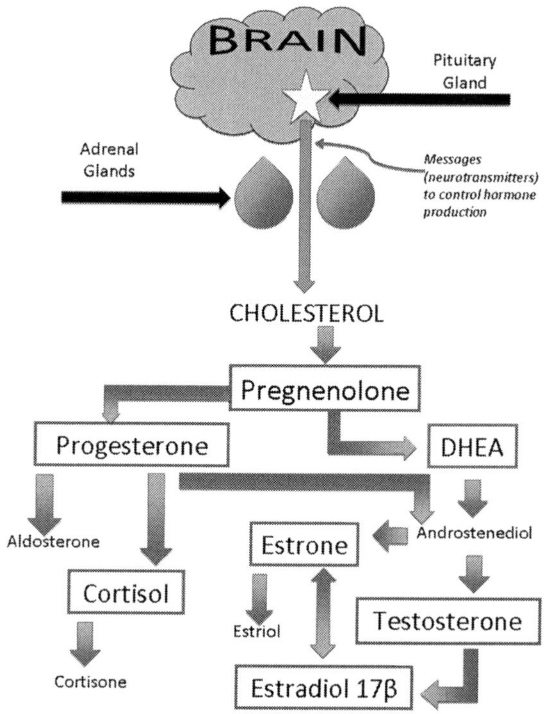

As mentioned earlier, hormones travel all through the body, either in the blood or in the fluid around the cells. The hormones are looking for *target* cells. An easy way to understand the relationship hormones have with target cells is to think of hormones as messengers and target cells as recipients of their deliveries. If the messengers were working for a company that is building an entire city, for example, they would be responsible for the delivery of all the blueprints and plans for implementing the city's infrastructure. In other words, target cells are the primary destinations for the hormones that are busily searching for the right target cells for their deliveries. Target cells check each and every hormonal delivery to determine if it has arrived in the right place or if it needs to move on to another target cell to make contact. When the right "blueprints" are delivered to the right places, all the "workers" inside the city—the body—begin to carry out the plans tailored for them. Some of these hormonal messengers travel very short distances and some are required to travel all over the body, but each has its own unique set of plans and directions to deliver. In addition to the distance they travel, some hormones reach a large variety of target cells, and some only a very specific few. The key is that only the target cells that are made to receive the precise hormone that arrives can respond to that hormone. If and when the hormone is accepted, it triggers a cascade of reactions inside the target cells that affect the associated bodily functions.

Let's take our city analogy a step further as an example. In this city, all the target cells will need to have access to the plans for the electrical wiring so that all the houses and businesses will have power. Therefore, the messengers (hormones) carrying the electrical information will have to deliver the plans to all these locations.

When it comes to plumbing all the buildings in our city, there will be many different needs. Is it a house or a commercial property? Does old plumbing have to be updated or does new plumbing require installation? Is the need basic, such as a sink and a toilet, or more complicated, with showers, bathtubs, washing machines, refrigerators, and so on? The messengers (hormones) carrying the correct information need to get to the correct locations to fulfill the exact specifications. This is why the precise nature of the delivery process—whether in a city or in the body—is so important.

Fat-based and water-based hormones

Another important thing about hormones is that they fall into two categories: *fat-based* and *water-based.* This is significant because all cells are essentially made up of fatty shells. Just think of a cell as a balloon. Picture this balloon with two layers of fat, one layer on the outside and one on the inside. These layers together make up the balloon's (cell's) wall, or its membrane. Because hormones like progesterone, estrogen, and testosterone are fat-based, they can move easily through the cell's membrane, which is also fat-based. However, these same fat-based hormones have more difficulty maneuvering in the bloodstream because of the blood's high water content. The body has special protein hormones, called "peptides," that function in the precise capacity of escorting these hormones wherever they need to go.

One of the most common peptides is insulin, which we discussed earlier. Others include: the growth hormone (GH), the luteinizing hormone (LH), and the follicle-stimulating hormone (FSH), all involved in a woman's monthly cycle and pregnancy; prolactin, responsible for stimulating milk production in pregnant women; and glucocorticoids, which help with immune function as well as the breakdown of glucose (sugar) for energy and the breakdown of fat. This scenario is reversed for all the water-based hormones, since water-based hormones can maneuver easily in the bloodstream but have a hard time penetrating the two layers of fat around the membrane of the cell.

Natural hormones made by the body function like locks and keys or puzzle pieces, as in the diagram on the next page. The "R," or "receptor," end fits perfectly into a cell receptor to "unlock" whatever process or action is supposed to take place. The other end of the puzzle piece, the "E," or "enzyme," end fits exactly into enzymes that change one type of hormone into another type of hormone for the body to use or make into a form that can be excreted.

Don't forget: enzymes are molecules (our tiny bubbles) that speed up the rate of chemical reactions inside cells. They are the traffic cops directing the traffic that flows in different directions at different speeds, so that everything gets exactly where it needs to go as quickly as possible.

Natural Hormones.

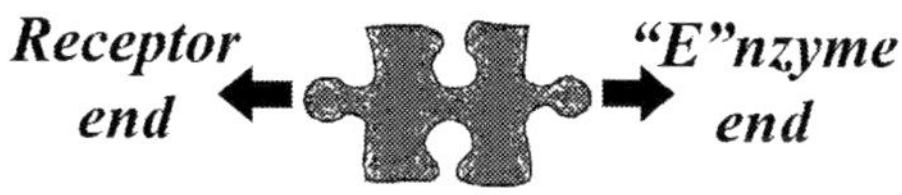

With a subject as complex as hormones it is almost impossible to keep it simple without oversimplifying it to the point where the explanation loses meaning. Therefore, my goal is to supply just enough facts to make the information here pertinent and memorable. To suggest that these brief explanations cover all there is to know would be like saying men and women understand all there is to know about each other—and we know that will never happen. The only thing we can do is keep learning. With that said, so far we've discussed enough about hormones and what they do that you probably realize that countless complex processes are taking place in your body every second of every minute of every hour of every day of every year of your life. But don't try to understand all of it. No one does. Just understand and remember as much as you can, and apply what you learn so that you can better manage the things that come your way. Perhaps your newfound knowledge about hormones will help you experience fewer mood swings, fewer or lighter cramps, diminished, fewer, or the cessation of headaches, less weight gain, or more energy. Who knows?

Synthetic/manufactured hormones

Synthetic hormones are manufactured to look like the ones our bodies produce naturally. *Synthetic*, according to the *Merriam-Webster* dictionary, means "devised, arranged, or fabricated for special situations to imitate or replace usual realities; the composition or combination of parts or elements so as to form a whole; the production of a substance by the union of chemical elements, groups, or simpler compounds or by the degradation of a complex compound." However, so far scientists have not found a way to produce synthetic hormones to match our natural ones precisely. What typically happens in the production process is that an additional chemical bond or molecule is added to the base animal or plant hormone to make it "unique." If the label of "unique" can be applied, that hormone can now be patented by the company producing it. The most controversial synthetic hormones ever manufactured are those that use pregnant mare urine, as found in the drug Premarin®, for example. Regrettably, while the hormone found in mare urine is natural to mares, it is not natural to humans, and has been proven to cause cancer, cardiovascular disease, and death.

When a manufactured (synthetic) hormone enters a cell receptor, the "R" end will be *similar*, but not a perfect fit. It's like trying to force one wrong puzzle piece into another where it doesn't really belong. Though it may appear identical in shape, color, and size to the piece you need and you might get it to fit if you try hard enough, forcing it only throws off all the other pieces around it. That one incorrectly placed piece will have a ripple effect and cause all the others to lose their ability to fit exactly and ultimately the entire picture will not appear as intended. The same can happen to your body when an unnatural hormone ("wrong" piece) is used instead of a natural hormone ("correct" piece), and this can create many possible side effects.

Synthetic Hormones.

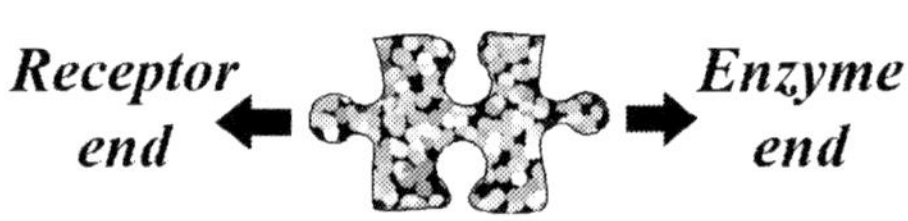

The "E," or "enzyme," end of a synthetic hormone is not an identical match with the body's self-produced hormones either. When this is the case, the hormone may not undergo the desired transformation into another hormone or be properly broken down and excreted from the body. When the hormone cannot be integrated appropriately, it will often end up stored in the body's fat. As we know, this result can keep the body from working the way it should and create more side effects as well.

The Prempro® fiasco

One of the most significant and hideous examples of the use of a synthetic hormone combination gone awry was revealed in 2002 in a published study of the Women's Health Initiative (WHI). In this case, the National Institutes of Health sponsored what was intended to be a long-term research study to assess the safety and effectiveness of estrogen in the form of pregnant horse urine and progestin, synthetic progesterone, when they were taken together in the form of a pill called Prempro®. The study's participants were women ages 50 to 79 who were to be followed for the most common causes of death, disability, and poor quality of life—that is, cardiovascular disease, cancer, and osteoporosis—in postmenopausal women. The researchers of this study wanted to determine if taking the combined synthetic estrogen and progestin would help prevent heart disease and decrease the number of hip fractures in the participants.

This study was originally designed to run for 8.5 years. It was abruptly terminated after 5 years, however, when the researchers saw that their hypothesis was wrong. Horribly, not only did they find a *26% increase* in breast cancer in the women who received the hormones compared with the women who received a placebo, or sugar pill, but they also saw a *29% increase* in heart attacks and a *22% increase* in total cardiovascular disease!

Dr. Dominique Toran-Allerand, professor of anatomy and cell biology at Columbia University, shared the following retrospective information in the *New York Times* about this study: "The WHI Study on estrogen-progestin replacement was doomed from the beginning, since the biology of the hormones and their receptors does not seem to have been considered in the design of the clinical trial. Premarin®, the estrogen used in this trial, is a complex mixture of horse estrogens, along with other steroids not normally found in women. Provera®, the progestin used, is a synthetic analog of the normal hormone progesterone. Progestins like Provera® block the beneficial actions of estrogen and may have harmful effects of their own by binding to receptors of other steroid hormones."

In reviewing numerous opinions and comments associated with this study, many doctors and others within the medical community seem to agree that this outcome was not entirely unexpected as there had been a noticeable increase in the type of symptoms referenced in the study even in the 10 years *preceding* the WHI study.

Unsurprisingly, the results of this study on Premarin® started a virtual panic among women taking any type of hormone replacement therapy and hormones in general. Women began looking for other alternatives to mitigate their symptoms and to try to avoid the negative and potentially deadly side effects of the hormone therapy the study had incorporated. This shift in thinking about how to treat some hormone-related issues set off a firestorm of activity and controversy. Many women stopped the hormone therapy they were using immediately, even if it had nothing to do with the WHI trials. Prominent women within the medical community made it very public that they were removing themselves and all family members from hormonal therapy.

Premarin® has been in use since 1942. What is surprising is that even after the alarming findings of the WHI study, this drug, which has already been proven dangerous, is still being used to treat women for hot flashes and other symptoms of menopause and "hormonal imbalance." For over 60 years physicians prescribed Premarin® and countless women took it because no one challenged its safety or effectiveness—until the WHI study. This is a glaring example that drugs that have been "approved" are not necessarily safe, and that just because a lot of people are using it does not mean it is any less risky. I refer to this kind of decision-making as The Sheep Principle. Sheep do what the majority of other sheep are doing; they go with the leader. You've heard the story about how if one sheep plunges to its death by jumping off of a cliff, all the other sheep follow mindlessly to meet the same fate. Don't be a sheep. If you insist on being a sheep, be the lead sheep, so at least you can see where you are going. Being in the back of the flock obstructs your view and puts you in a decidedly compromised position.

Again, do not be misled into taking a drug just because a doctor suggests it or because you've seen ads on television about the miraculous results you'll get by using it. The Women's Health Initiative study proves this point in spades, where women served as guinea pigs for a drug that had not been researched thoroughly prior to its use.

How many of us have heard our parents say, "Just because your friend jumps off the bridge, does that mean you're going to jump off too?" This is one of the many lessons we may prefer to ignore because we think *we* know best. But in the end, it's always best to think for ourselves and make informed decisions, even if it means swimming against the tide.

16

Bioidentical Hormones

We've discussed synthetic hormones, what they are, how they're made, and how dangerous they can be. It's time now to transition to a more positive topic, that of *bioidentical* hormones. If you haven't heard much about bioidentical hormones yet, you likely will soon because massive amounts of information have recently been surfacing about them, particularly since the WHI report was made public.

Many doctors have been prescribing bioidentical hormones for 20 to 30 years. Actress and author Suzanne Somers made a huge impact on the public's consciousness when she brought bioidentical hormones to the public's attention with her bestselling book, *The Sexy Years*, which provided a wealth of information regarding hormones and menopause. Lately there has also been much discussion on *Oprah*, *The Doctors*, and other popular TV shows that has contributed to making bioidenticals much more widely understood.

What's the buzz all about? Let's investigate.

Bioidentical hormones are derived from plants, primarily soybeans and wild Mexican yams. Hormones that come from plants are also referred to as *phytoestrogens* and are very similar in structure to the ones that are produced naturally in the body. It is because bioidenticals have such a similar structure to naturally produced hormones that they are believed to be able to function without the negative and potentially deadly side effects of synthetic hormones. It is important to note that even though these hormones from plants—the phytoestrogens—must be transformed to create "identical" counterparts to those already in the body, they are still not considered "synthetic" in the negative sense of the word.

As previously defined, "synthetic" is the combining of parts or elements to form a whole. This definition can be applied to bioidenticals as well, as they are "synthesized," or changed, into a form the body can use. The difference is that when they are changed or combined, bioidenticals become exact replicas of the body's own hormones.

Compounding hormones

You may not be familiar with the term "compounded" even if you know about bioidentical hormones due to their recent gain in popularity. Basically, because traditional, non-compounded, manufactured hormones are produced with a one-size-fits-all approach, this model often fails to meet the unique requirements of each individual and a different approach is required. Compounding pharmacies make it possible to get just what the individual needs by mixing formulas in specific strengths, quantities, and combinations. In some instances, when an original manufacturer is no longer producing a particular drug, a compounding pharmacy also has the means to create the same discontinued product.

One significant reason why people prefer compounding pharmacies and their products is that manufactured drugs often use additives, such as gluten and preservatives, that can cause allergic reactions. Another important advantage of compounded, or customized, medications is the variety of dosage forms available. In regards to bioidentical hormone replacement therapy, there are distinct advantages to dosage forms that bypass the digestive tract and liver, where significant amounts of the drugs are often broken down before reaching the bloodstream itself. Examples of these compounded drug forms are nasal sprays, drops that are placed under the tongue (called "sublingual"), and/or suppositories for those individuals who are unable to swallow.

In addition to size and strength concerns, there are also times when a medicine tastes unpalatable. As an adult, you can probably force yourself to take it because you understand how it will benefit you, but kids don't rationalize the way we do and usually refuse to take something if it tastes bad. In this case, a compounding pharmacist may be able to add something to the prescription to flavor or sweeten it for the child's consumption.

Many pharmacies have the ability to combine, or compound, ingredients to a very limited capacity. But when compounded prescriptions require more in-depth combining, compounding pharmacies have more extensive and specialized equipment as well as pharmacists who have received additional training for the specialized practice of mixing plant-derived hormones for the patient's use (with a doctor's prescription).

Interestingly, even though compounding requires more equipment and education, the cost of a compounded prescription is generally less than the typical bulk, manufactured option. A great resource for information regarding compounding pharmacies is the Pharmacy Compounding Accreditation Board (PCAB) at www.pcab.info, and you can read more about compounding pharmacies at www.hormonebasics.com.

But now let's return for a moment to the subject of bioidenticals and the devastating outcome of the WHI study. It was because the outcome of this study was so overwhelmingly negative that a hurried search began for a hormone alternative, and it was through this search that many women found bioidentical hormones to be an option. There still seems to be a lot of confusion when discussing natural and bioidentical hormones, however. I believe much of the confusion comes from the fact that the two terms are often used interchangeably even though their meanings are actually quite different.

To validate this opinion, I looked for a dictionary definition of "bioidentical" in two medical dictionaries, but neither had the word listed. With that said, if we pull the word apart I think we can achieve a pretty credible definition. The word "bio" is defined as "life" by *Mosby's Medical Dictionary*; *Taber's Cyclopedic Medical Dictionary* defines "bio" as "relationship to life." The word "identical" is pretty self-explanatory: "the same." So, it would be safe to say that we could define bioidentical as "the same as life," or, in this instance, the same as it naturally occurs in the body.

The *Merriam-Webster* dictionary is not a medical dictionary, but includes "bioidentical," defining it as "possessing identical molecular structure, especially in relation to an endogenously produced substance." *Endogenous* means growing or produced inside the body. For simplicity's sake, we will refer to your self-made hormones as "natural" and the ones from plants as "bioidentical."

At the time the WHI study results were made public, the companies who had been producing bioidentical hormones heard the outcry for an option to the synthetic versions and saw the opportunity their plant-based products offered. Even though some doctors and patients had been reaping the benefits of bioidenticals for years, this time really stands out as the birth of the bioidentical boom. The medical community as a whole soon responded by advising consumers of the potential dangers of the now ever-more-popular bioidenticals. It's not surprising, therefore, that the public remains confused by all the mixed signals and conflicting information propagated by the scientific and medical industries about whether bioidenticals are good or bad.

Here is what I want you to know. The only way to get true, non-suspect, bioidenticals is from a legitimate, trustworthy compounding pharmacy. To do so you need a prescription from a doctor. And although there are doctors who prescribe them, many do not, and many are not advocates for their use. Furthermore, there is an obvious division in the medical community on this matter and it is possible that even your medical doctor is as confused as you are.

First, doctors are often told that a drug like Premarin®, the one used in the WHI study, works—and that it is still a viable prescribing option. In Premarin®'s case, these doctors have been told for over 65 years about this drug's superior qualities and benefits. This kind of misinformation can be hard to unlearn. It is also not unusual for doctors to be bombarded with information on the benefits of the drugs on the market and the benefits of prescribing them to their patients to the degree that the potential negative side effects are all but ignored when important decisions are being made. We should not forget that all the women in that widespread study with its horrific results had families and friends and that the suffering was widespread. That's why I have to ask: How many women who are looking for answers end up finding their lives and wellbeing destroyed at the expense of "research" and profits?

17

Your Doctor's Struggles & the Drug Companies

Our society has been indoctrinated to follow the directive of doctors and the pharmaceutical industry without question and has become accustomed to believing they offer the best, or possibly the only viable, option for whatever our presenting condition requires. Many of us take the prescriptions we are given or have the surgery performed as we are advised, assuming it is the best thing for us. Unfortunately, this is not always the case.

I believe the vast majority of doctors are doing their best to help each person under each set of unique circumstances. I know that physicians are given the best education possible to work in what I believe is the most difficult profession there is—that of caring for other human beings. The health, wellbeing, and life of every patient they see is in their hands. It may be hard for others to appreciate the sense of responsibility and the stress this work creates, but I would imagine the providers' families, who share in the burden as well, would agree.

Most doctors do their job, confident in the education they have received and knowing that while patients' conditions may remain relatively the same, the way to treat them and the options available change all the time. New drugs and procedures are introduced almost daily, each one said to be an improvement on the last. In terms of drugs alone, I have lost track of how many prescription drug ads I see on television and in print.

Perhaps it is true that if you take the drug you see in the ad you will spend more time laughing with your girlfriends or sitting in a bathtub on the beach with your significant other and gazing at the sunset. Perhaps, as Dr. Wayne Dyer has said with sarcasm, you have a real need to go clamming with your dog or on a road trip with the guys. But by focusing your attention on these appealing scenarios, the drug companies are hoping we will overlook the numerous, potentially dangerous side-effects of the drugs being pushed at us. The idea is that the drugs will change your life; that you will be relaxed and happy if you use them. And because that's what most of us want, all we hear is that our life will be transformed if we, "Go to your doctor and ask if the drug is right for you." In the old days, we went to the doctor if we felt bad and a medicine might be prescribed. Nowadays, we go in demanding drugs we've seen on television because we want our lives to look like the scenes in the ads.

The drug craze

Unfortunately, with so many drugs flooding the market, doctors may not always get the opportunity to learn as much as the public that takes those drugs would like them to learn before prescribing them as "solutions" to their presenting problem(s). After graduation from medical school, much of a doctor's education about drugs used to treat specific conditions comes straight from the sales representatives who work for the drug companies. These sales representatives are well versed in selling the various drugs on the market, emphasizing the benefits and de-emphasizing the not-so-pleasant potential side effects. I know this to be true because I personally spent time as a pharmaceutical rep before going into chiropractic practice. What this means is that doctors may be relying solely on the accuracy and thoroughness of the information provided by the drug rep to make their determinations about prescribing certain drugs for their patients. Most doctors are too busy to thoroughly investigate and research even one or two drugs a week, let alone the number of new ones they are introduced to on what seems like an almost daily basis.

Contrary to popular belief, I believe the majority of doctors are overworked and underpaid. Medical practice is not the prestigious, highly lucrative profession it once may have been, unless a doctor specializes in a particular area and even then there are still no guarantees. Don't get me wrong, I think most do okay with their yearly salaries, but if you factor in the hours of work and the stress levels involved, I think there are many who think seriously about searching for a different career path.

In fact, according to a report by the Physicians' Foundation published in *Reuters* in November of 2008, most primary care doctors in the United States reported they felt overworked and nearly half said they planned to either cut back on how many patients they were seeing or quit medicine entirely. Specifically, 60% of 12,000 general practice physicians said they would not recommend medicine as a career; more than 90% said the time they devoted to non-clinical paperwork had increased in the last 3 years; and 63% said that time spent on paperwork has caused them to spend less time with each patient. Overall, 76% percent of physicians said they were working at "full capacity" or were "overextended and overworked."

I believe the majority of doctors act in good faith and with the best interests of their patients in mind in regards to the decisions they make about the drugs they use. I also think that most of the pharmaceutical sales reps act in good faith when presenting their material to the doctors. With that said, pharmaceutical reps are clearly under the directives of the companies they work for and they rely on these companies for accuracy, comprehensiveness, and specificity in regards to the information on the drugs they are peddling.

That leaves us with the drug companies. Once upon a time, before Big Pharma (as it is called) existed, I believe a group of intelligent, caring individuals got together to form the first company to truly help improve the health of their fellow humans through pharmacology. I would like to think it was more about the good they would do rather than the amount of money they would make. I like to think they did it because they believed they could make a difference in peoples' lives.

But, to be honest, I feel that somewhere along the way the drug companies got too big. In an obvious generalization, I'd say that though the leaders of these companies have great business minds for maximizing profits, their biggest concern has become the bottom line, not the safety, health, and wellbeing of the people using the drugs they manufacture. And remember, these "people" are all of us, every single one of us who pays for the drugs and for the insurance policies that we hope will help us purchase them. In my opinion, as the money started rolling in so quickly and in such big quantities it was the money that began to guide the direction and intent of the industry. And if the scientists testing the new drugs are paid by the pharmaceutical companies themselves, we have to ask ourselves just how reliable this information can possibly be.

The pharmaceutical industry has unquestionably saved countless lives. But it also must take responsibility for the loss of countless lives, intentional or otherwise. After all, knowledge and intent does not always determine outcome.

Bringing drugs to the market

Somewhere along the scientific, medical, and pharmaceutical path hormones and the need women have for them came onto the scene and the scientists, chemists, and other experts got busy formulating hormones as fast as they could to meet that need. But it is impossible to artificially recreate anything in a lab to be an exact duplicate in every aspect of its natural counterpart. Current scientific knowledge and technology gets closer and closer all the time and is the source of great hope. Unfortunately, the same knowledge and technology used inappropriately or without enough research behind it can be dangerous or deadly.

Replacement hormones were born directly from this perceived public need and through the wonders of science. These hormonal remedies were created, formulated, processed, and submitted to the government for approval to help millions of suffering women.

To bring a new drug to the market can easily cost hundreds of millions, possibly billions, of dollars these days and can take decades from inception of the drug's research to the end product. It is no secret that the two biggest reasons for the pharmaceutical industry's hesitation to try to bring more bioidenticals to market through FDA approval are time and money.

At the 17th Annual Meeting of The North American Menopause Society, James A. Simon, M.D. shared the following information as an example:

To obtain FDA approval for an estrogen drug, the manufacturer must conduct at least one and usually two randomized, prospective, placebo-controlled clinical trials. To obtain an indication to treat a specific condition, the drug must meet clinical requirements that support the indication. To be indicated for treatment of hot flashes, for instance, a drug must be statistically superior to the placebo in reducing both the frequency and severity of hot-flash symptoms. To establish superiority, a manufacturer must provide 12 weeks of data demonstrating the safety and efficacy of its drug in decreasing the number of moderate to severe hot flashes, defined as 56 or more occurrences per week per patient. Also, the drug must reduce the number of hot flashes per day by at least two. Superior efficacy compared with placebo must be evident within four weeks after study initiation. In addition, a manufacturer must establish the lowest effective dose to alleviate symptoms. Along with documentation of safety and efficacy outcomes, other study requirements include tracking levels of lipids, lipoproteins, and coagulation factors and monitoring serum levels of active, and in some cases inactive, metabolites. Only after meeting all of these criteria can such a drug be indicated for the treatment of hot flashes as intended.

Requirements for approval of progestogens are even more complicated because of health risks that became evident in several clinical trials that took place. Manufacturers must conduct an endometrial hyperplasia (a condition of excessive proliferation of the cells of the endometrium, or inner lining of the uterus) prevention study of at least 12 months' duration, but often up to 24 months. The acceptable rate of hyperplasia is 1% or less with a confidence interval that does not exceed 4% for the population.

The FDA requires all manufactured Hormone Therapy (HT) products to be labeled and to include warning language, but compounded Bioidentical Hormone Therapy (BHT) products are typically not labeled and do not include warnings. This is not true for quality-oriented pharmacies that are accredited by the PCAB, however, and that are required to include warnings and patient information with each product provided. Paradoxically, all manufactured estrogen products must include the following warning language related to endometrial cancer risk: "There is no evidence that the use of 'natural' estrogens results in a different endometrial risk profile than 'synthetic estrogens' of equivalent estrogen dose."

BHT proponents who claim their estrogen products are "natural" and not synthetic do not carry this warning. The FDA requires additional warning language for HT based on the WHI study results that demonstrated an increased risk of myocardial infarction, stroke, pulmonary embolism, deep vein thrombosis, and invasive breast cancer in certain populations, and warned that different combinations and dosage formulations of estrogens and progestogens had not been studied in the trial. According to the FDA, the risks are assumed to be similar.

In summary, it is through the search for and research of hormones and how they are made that bioidentical and synthetics hormones were discovered. Synthetic hormones are the ones manufactured, or chemically created, in a lab to produce a usable form. The companies that manufacture these synthetic hormones are legally permitted to own patents on them. Patented drugs are the ones that are the most lucrative for the pharmaceutical companies. If they can't patent a drug, they can't charge as much for it because the next "guy down the street" can manufacture the exact same thing. Of course, this is true in almost every industry.

The problem with a substance that is not patentable, like the hormones most people categorize as "natural," or "bioidentical," is that you can't really count on making a great deal of money from them. Since the pharmaceutical industry is without question driven by money (as well as what I hope is a desire to help people), they haven't really been interested in spending much money on the research or production of bioidentical hormones, at least on a scale to meet the current growing interest and need.

18

Prescription & Compounding Options

According to Goodman and Gilman's *The Pharmacological Basis of Therapeutics* (10th edition, McGraw-Hill, 2001), "Commercially manufactured hormone therapy is intended not to replace hormones but to relieve symptoms. Consumers may not know that several Hormone Therapy (HT) products approved by the U.S. Food and Drug Administration are structurally identical to hormones produced by the ovaries. In that regard, they are "bioidentical." Consumers also may be unaware that a "drug" may be defined as any chemical agent that affects living protoplasm, which therefore includes most substances, including Bioidentical Hormone Therapy, or BHT."

Prescription bioidentical estrogen and progesterone are available in FDA-approved hormone therapy products, including Estradiol®, Estrace®, the Climara® patch, the Vivelle-Dot® patch, and natural progesterone, which is sold as Prometrium®. Both the estrogen and progesterone found in these products are derived from plants and processed so the body can utilize them just as they do their compounded counterparts. FDA-approved bioidentical hormones have been tested for purity, potency, safety, and concentration, so that if a woman needs one of the limited dosage options available, their quality should produce a predictable outcome.

The likely reason these FDA-approved hormones are not used as often as the bioidenticals from compounding pharmacies is that they are dispensed in generalized doses; in other words, in a one-size-fits-all form. Hormones in the compounded form, on the other hand, can be modified in terms of specific amounts and individual doses to better suit each unique individual.

Bioidentical hormones have gone through a conversion process before they are used by a compounding pharmacy. It is for this reason that many oppose the use of bioidentical hormones, saying that they undergo a conversion process that keeps them from being "natural" and thus puts them in the same category as synthetics. It is true that bioidenticals have to be converted or modified in order for the body to use them most effectively. You can't stroll through a soybean or wild yam patch, casually chewing on the plants as you go, for example, and expect to reap any hormonal benefit. It doesn't work that way. But bioidenticals are *not* the same as synthetic hormones.

Pharmaceutical compounding

Purity, quality, potency, safety, and consistency are at the heart of the argument by the majority of those against the bioidenticals being marketed and used today. According to the North American Menopause Society (NAMS), "Custom compounds may provide certain benefits, such as individualized doses and mixtures of products and forms that aren't available commercially. However, they may also pose risks to consumers. These compounds haven't been approved by the Food and Drug Administration (FDA) and as a result haven't been tested for purity, potency, efficacy, or safety. These products may even contain unknown contaminants. For this reason, NAMS does not recommend these custom-mixed products over well-tested, government approved commercial products for the majority of women." It is important to note that, according to the PCAB, all of its accredited quality-oriented compounding pharmacies test all of their ingredients for purity and potency. Purity is the indicator of the grade of ingredients used and a "certificate of analysis" confirms the purity grade. Potency is determined by an independent laboratory analysis.

The Center for Drug Evaluation Research defines pharmaceutical compounding as "the combining, mixing, or altering of ingredients to create a customized medication for an individual patient in response to a licensed practitioner's prescription. Compounding does not generally include mixing or reconstituting commercial products in accordance with the manufacturer's instructions or the product's approved labeling. The quality of a finished compounded drug product can be affected by numerous factors, including the quality of the active pharmaceutical ingredient used and the compounding practices of the pharmacy in which the product is created."

According to the Center for Drug Evaluation and Research (CDER) (at www.fda.gov/drugs/default.htm), since 1990 the FDA has become aware of more than 55 product quality problems associated with compounded products, many of which have resulted in product recalls. It is very important to remember, however, that the compounding pharmacies in this study were "limited to those permitting Internet purchase of the drug products chosen for sampling," and that there were only 12 pharmacies included in this small study.

In this survey by the FDA's Division of Prescription Drug Compliance and Surveillance in 2001, 29 product samples made by 12 online compounding pharmacies were reviewed, including hormonal compounds, antibiotics, steroids, anesthetics, and drugs to treat glaucoma, asthma, iron-deficiency anemia, and erectile dysfunction in various forms of dosage, such as pills, injectables, and inhalants. Ten, or 34% of these 29 sampled products failed one or more standard quality tests performed, and 9 of those 10 products failed tests for potency. All of the sampled products that failed potency analyses had sub-potent results, indicating that the products analyzed contained less of the active ingredient(s) than expected and as were described in the product's label.

Each year, the FDA routinely samples drug products made by commercial manufacturers and analyzes these samples in FDA laboratories. More than 3,000 drug products from commercial manufacturers have been sampled and analyzed by FDA since 1996. The failure rate for commercially produced samples has been less than 2%. When compared to this failure rate, the percentage of sampled compounded products failing analytical testing in this survey, that is, 34%, was higher than expected.

Some of the biggest concerns that can be raised relative to the FDA's study focus on the chain of custody, storage, and timely laboratory analysis of the compounds in question. For example, if a sample sits in the glove box of a car or in the light of an office window for days or weeks before it is sent to the lab, in all likelihood it will have undergone some level of deterioration. The general public has been led to believe that any results that come from a lab are not to be questioned. But for the FDA's analytical lab to correctly test and guarantee the accuracy of the tests of the drugs in the study, not only would the samples have had to arrive in a timely and efficient manner, but the researchers would have had to know the additional ingredients in the formulas. In point of fact, the FDA's labs did not have this information.

If you begin to pay attention to the true limitations of "FDA approval" and what that means for the "safety" of the products tested, you will see that many of them, though they may be both "approved" and labeled "safe" for consumption, are neither.

Again, bear in mind that this survey had several major limitations, including a small sample size, the inability to collect and complete original and repeat analyses on all product samples originally identified, and the fact that the compounding pharmacies selected for the survey were limited to those permitting Internet purchase of the drug products chosen for sampling. Despite these limitations, however, this survey provides valuable, preliminary information on the quality of selected compounded drug products currently marketed and the findings highlight the importance of carefully and properly compounding drug products to minimize risks to consumers.

It is also important to take heed of the FDA's warning that, as with any other profession, there are good practices and not-so-good, or even bad, practices. This is why if you are considering using bioidenticals, find a credible, reliable, proven, and trustworthy compounding pharmacy. Recognize that some of the best compounding pharmacies in the country are on line and allow for on-line refills, so you can be assured that pharmacies with websites are not necessarily any less credible or trustworthy. The compounding industry has taken measures to ensure the highest quality product for safety and effectiveness. Great practices and procedures help produce great products that in turn help produce a great response. As mentioned earlier, if you have questions regarding compounding pharmacies or their practices, the Pharmacy Compounding Accreditation Board is the best resource I have found.

Even though the bioidenticals associated with compounding pharmacies haven't been submitted to or approved by the FDA, this doesn't mean there is no accountability by the pharmacies that distribute them. It is also important to remember that although compounded medications do not require FDA approval, they are not considered experimental or investigational. The FDA clearly states that "Compounding is part of the practice of pharmacy/medicine."

There are actually several entities that oversee the actions of compounding pharmacies and the enforcement of pharmacy compounding standards is the responsibility of state pharmacy boards. The United States Pharmacopeia (USP) sets the standards regarding mixing. Other agencies that are involved are the Drug Enforcement Agency (DEA), the Occupational Safety and Health Administration (OSHA), the Environmental Protection Agency (EPA), and the Nuclear Regulatory Agency (NRC). In addition to government agencies, there are numerous state and national pharmacy boards that create their own rules and regulations.

In 2004, eight pharmacy organizations established the Pharmacy Compounding Accreditation Board , or PCAB, to establish high quality standards for compounding pharmacies. They are: the American College of Apothecaries, the American Pharmacists Association, the International Academy of Compounding Pharmacists, the National Association of Boards of Pharmacy, the National Community Pharmacists Association, the National Council of State Pharmacy Association Executives, the National Home Infusion Association, and the United States Pharmacopeia Convention (USP).

Compounding pharmacies can voluntarily submit an application, but must meet extremely strict requirements before they are approved. The Pharmacy Compounding Accreditation Board indicates that it "saw a need for an enhanced, profession-wide system of standards by which each compounding pharmacy [could] test its quality processes. Compounding pharmacists also wanted a mechanism to allow them to know that [a pharmacy's] quality is high and that their patients are as safe as possible. PCAB Accreditation gives patients and prescribers a way to select a pharmacy that meets high quality standards."

I highly recommend finding a compounding pharmacy that has been certified as Pharmacy Compounding Accreditation Board-approved. This is one way you can help assure yourself you are getting the highest quality of product from a reputable, trustworthy compounding pharmacy.

19

Compounded Hormones

You now know there are FDA-approved bioidentical estrogen and progesterone products and bioidentical products that have not been approved by the FDA and are available only by prescription through a compounding pharmacy. Compounded estrogen hormones come in different forms and include *estradiol*, *esterified*, *estropipate*, and *micronized*. We'll look briefly at each type.

Estradiol estrogen is derived from soybeans and/or wild yams and is structurally the same as the estrogen made in the body. Estradiol is the predominate form naturally found in the body.

Esterified estrogens can also be derived from soybeans and wild yams, but usually have higher levels of estrone and lower levels of estrogen than estradiol estrogen. Esterified estrogens have been found to increase the risk of developing endometrial hyperplasia, a condition that may lead to cancer of the uterine lining.

Estropipate estrogen can also be derived from plant sources. Its synthetic form, called Ogen®, is described in the manufacturer's literature as "prepared from purified crystalline estrone" and "stabilized with Piperazine®." Piperazine® is a compound used in the treatment of worm infections. A quick search on the Internet will show you Piperazine® is most commonly used in pet de-wormers. I've never understood the appeal—or need—for balancing hormones and getting rid of worms with the same treatment!

Micronized estrogen is made from soybeans. "Micronized" means it is made so the estrogen is reduced into small enough components that it can be absorbed in the bloodstream before the stomach and digestive system can break it down and possibly affect its potency.

Use of any natural or synthetic hormone should be discussed thoroughly with your health care provider for a number of very important reasons. First of all, as previously mentioned, just because something is "natural" doesn't mean it is good for you and secondly, too much of a good thing can be bad. Make sure your doctor is aware of any other drug you are taking. Some common prescription drugs, such as erythromycin and clarithromycin, may affect hormone levels or have other adverse reactions. These antibiotics are frequently used to treat certain infections caused by bacteria, such as bronchitis, pertussis (whooping cough), pneumonia, ear, sinus, intestine, lung, urinary tract, and skin infections, ulcers, and venereal disease. They are also used prophylactically, before some surgery and dental work to prevent infection.

Other drugs that may affect hormone levels include Ketoconazole® and Itraconazole®, most often used to treat infections that can spread to different parts of the body through the bloodstream. These include yeast infections of the mouth, throat, skin, urinary tract, and blood, and fungal infections that affect the fingernails and/or toenails, as well as those that start on the skin or in the lungs and can spread through the body. If, for whatever reason, you don't want to or can't ask your doctor, ask your pharmacist. Pharmacists specialize in drugs and they are the ones with extensive knowledge. In my experience, if they don't have the answer, they are always more than happy to get it for you.

To summarize: A natural hormone is one your body makes on its own; a bioidentical hormone is an exact structural replica of your natural hormone, derived from a plant and converted for your body to use; and a synthetic hormone is artificially created by humans in a lab through the use of chemicals. Synthetic hormones are similar to your natural hormones, but pose the threat of numerous side effects.

Now that we've talked about the different sources of hormones, in the next chapter we'll move on to specific hormones, called *primary* hormones.

20

Primary Hormones

Of the more than 50 hormones that have been scientifically identified, there are four considered "primary" that we will discuss here: estrogen, progesterone, testosterone, and DHEA. We will also talk about cortisol, the "fight or flight" hormone, which has a powerful impact on the body, on health, and quite possibly on how much we enjoy the lives we live. As with all the primary hormones, an imbalance can cause a wide range of symptoms. Since the purpose of this book is to keep information simple, I have chosen to focus on the primary role each hormone plays and which ones can have the greatest affect.

Estrogen

Many people think of estrogen as one hormone when it is actually a term used for a group of hormones comprised of human estrogens, plant or phytoestrogens, animal estrogens, synthetic estrogens, and *eco-* or *xenoestrogens.*

There are three major types of estrogens found in humans: *estradiol*, the strongest; *estrone*, strong, but less strong than estradiol; and *estriol*, the weakest of the estrogens. Estradiol and estrone are considered to be the strong estrogens because they have shown a high potential to cause abnormal cell growth or cancer. Fortunately, estriol, the so-called "weak" estrogen, though primarily present only during pregnancy, helps balance cell growth and regulate the other two potential cancer-causing types of estrogens.

As you may recall from the lengthy list at the beginning of this book, hormones serve many vital functions in the body, most importantly in their role as neurotransmitters, chemicals that transmit nerve impulses from cell to cell. Furthermore, as you may also remember, based on the fact that each of these cells has a negative and positive charge, we can say that life forms are essentially made of and held together by energy. If you experience a large enough decrease in the chemicals required to support this electrical network of neurotransmitters, you may also experience symptoms such as a decrease in your energy levels, increased aches and pains, depression, increased irritability, anxiety, sensitivity to pain, eating disorders, and/or a disruption of your normal sleep rhythms…just to name a few.

Second, estrogens are responsible for promoting cell growth. It is this characteristic that can make them so dangerous. When estrogens operate uncontrollably so that cells grow or reproduce too quickly , cancerous conditions can develop. Kept in check and in proper balance, however, estrogens are not only beneficial, but crucial, to the body's many processes.

Third, estrogens are responsible for the proper formation and development of the female sex organs as well as the secondary sex characteristics. "Secondary sex characteristics" include breast development, the increase and/or redistribution of fat in specific areas, such as the thighs, buttocks, and hips, a widening of the hips (as a precursor to childbirth), and the onset of pubic and underarm hair growth.

Another major purpose of this group of estrogens is controlling the function of the uterus, especially as it pertains to menstrual cycles and preparation for possible pregnancy. In this case, estrogen is responsible for the development of the nutrient and blood-rich lining necessary for the egg's implantation. This is the lining shed during the monthly cycle in the event there is no implantation of a fertilized egg.

Estrogens are formed primarily by the ovaries and to some extent by the adrenal glands. Estrogens stimulate secondary sexual characteristics and have effects throughout the entire body, including the growth and maturation of long bones. Estrogen hormones, which control the course of the menstrual cycle, are also utilized therapeutically in any disorder that is attributable to estrogen deficiency or associated with estrogen therapy, such as menstrual disorders and menopausal problems.

Estradiol

Estradiol is the strongest, most predominate estrogen. Produced by the ovaries, its levels are known to decline dramatically at the time of menopause, when menstruation ceases. Also known as 17-beta estradiol, it is considered the most "active" form of estrogen as it is most often associated with increased energy, better moods, better memory, an increased ability to concentrate, an improved insulin response, normalized blood pressure, optimal bone density, better quality of sleep, a better sex drive, and a healthy, active metabolic rate, plus a number of other qualities.

One of the big problems with a decline in estradiol for any reason is that it can contribute to a decrease in the production of a hormone called *serotonin.* About 90% of all serotonin is found in the intestinal tract and is responsible for helping to control appetite, anger, body temperature, aggression, mood, sleep, metabolism, and sex drive. It is easy to see that if your hormones are not balanced and working as they should, your food cravings could go through the roof—not just because cravings often occur as a by-product of a hormonal imbalance, but also because of the effect of serotonin on this particular bodily function.

Serotonin itself is also a neurotransmitter and probably most widely known as a chemical that affects mood. Most prescription drugs to treat mood-related disorders are made to affect serotonin levels. It is probably no coincidence that so many women continually battle both mood and intestinal issues, given that the hormone serotonin plays such a big role in both. Because the body is so complex and has so many interacting functions, however, fixing this problem isn't always as easy as simply increasing or decreasing serotonin levels. It can be a major factor, though, and one that needs to be addressed in an effort to achieve overall balance.

Estrone

Estrone, the mid-strength estrogen produced primarily in the ovaries, is also produced in fat tissue. In women who have not yet experienced menopause, over 50% of all estrogen produced is made in the ovaries. After menopause, although estrone's production ceases in the ovaries and continues to be produced only in peripheral, or fat, tissue, it still remains the most abundant hormone. This predominance of estrone leads to the slower metabolism and the gain in body fat that many women experience during and after menopause or after a hysterectomy (surgery to remove the uterus). Estrone is also associated with a higher risk for breast and uterine cancers. Estrone's unique characteristic is its ability to be easily converted into the strongest form of estrogen, estradiol, for use in the body.

Estriol

Estriol is the weakest estrogen. Estriol is produced primarily by the placenta, a temporary organ formed during pregnancy that joins the mother and fetus and transfers oxygen and nutrients from the mother to the fetus. Estriol is found only in small amounts in non-pregnant women and its levels don't change to any significant degree after menopause. Estriol is referred to as the "safe" estrogen because it helps regulate estrone and estradiol, both of which can cause cancer.

Research suggests that estriol can help improve bone density, heart health, symptoms of multiple sclerosis, postmenopausal urinary tract health, and symptoms of menopause, such as vaginal dryness and hot flashes. Estriol supplementation appears to have all the benefits of estradiol and estrone and significantly fewer side effects.

It is interesting to note that as important as estriol is, there is very little discussion about it and, to my knowledge, no pharmaceutical company in the United States manufactures it. Estriol is not even found in the *Physician's Desk Reference*, or PDR, the book physicians utilize for information on both prescription and over-the-counter drugs (including recommended dosages, side effects, possible food and drug interactions, and detailed instructions for their use). Estriol is available for purchase, however, as a quick search on the Internet will show.

21

Estrogen & Symptoms of Imbalance

We've talked about how estrogens are responsible for hundreds of crucial functions in the brain and throughout the body and about the benefits and potential problems related to estrogen or an imbalance in its level. The list below reveals the extensive role estrogen plays in the body.

Estrogen:

- increases body fat, especially in hips, abdomen and thighs
- affects emotions, mood, pain perception, attentiveness, memory, energy, ambition, sleep
- helps skin stay soft and heal faster
- promotes hydration of tissues
- stimulates brain function
- increases HDL (good cholesterol)
- lowers LDL (bad cholesterol)

- helps prevent cholesterol deposits
- slows bone loss
- regulates body temperature
- promotes uterine lining and breast tissue growth
- creates progesterone receptors
- helps expand blood vessels
- stimulates the egg follicle in the ovary
- stops the growth of long bones when puberty begins
- helps maintain the lining of blood vessels
- inhibits factors involved with hardening of the arteries
- confers female secondary sex characteristics

Symptoms of estrogen deficiency include:

- depression, mood swings
- poor memory
- dry skin
- bladder infections
- headaches/migraines
- decreased sexual response, breast size, and stamina
- insomnia; sleep conditions
- osteoporosis, cardiovascular disease
- dry eyes/sinus conditions
- vaginal dryness, infections
- hot flashes, night sweats
- loss of ambition/drive

Symptoms of estrogen excess include:

- weight gain
- emotional hypersensitivity, depression, anger, agitation, irritability
- cold hands and feet
- headaches/migraines
- thyroid dysfunction
- insomnia
- water retention, bloating
- heavy bleeding, clotting
- cramping, breast tenderness, lumps, cysts, and enlargement
- decreased sexual response
- blood sugar instability
- irregular periods
- autoimmune disorders
- PCOS (Polycystic Ovary Syndrome), ovarian cysts, uterine fibroids
- copper toxicity
- breast cancer, endometrial cancer, uterine cancer

One possible additional symptom of estrogen excess is gall bladder dysfunction. The gall bladder is a small pear-shaped sac located under the liver that stores bile from the liver. Bile is a chemical made in and secreted by the liver. Bile's job is to break down fat into smaller particles, thereby aiding in its absorption and digestion in the small intestine. Bile also helps the body excrete waste products, including cholesterol, from the blood.

I have lost count of how many female patients, friends, and family members have had their gall bladders removed. Most men I know still have their gall bladders however, something that leads me to believe there is a major hormonal component to gall bladder function. Most of these women's cases are notable in the sense that they do not know why their gall bladders stopped functioning the way they were supposed to. But even more notable is the fact that in every single case, the only option offered to them was for its removal. Unfortunately, life does not return to "normal" after gall bladder removal. In fact, high-fat foods will often send anyone without a gall bladder into a tailspin.

To demonstrate, let's follow the track of a high-fat-content meal, any selection from the SAD diet we know so well. Let's look at what happens to a cheeseburger and fries, fried chicken, or tacos, when the primary organ that contains bile has been removed. Without this organ to store excess bile, the body is not as capable of breaking down the fat it has absorbed in the form of this food. If you don't have a gall bladder, some bile may be stored in the bile duct system, or "tubes," that transport bile to the small intestine. But where the big globs of fat were previously broken down into teeny tiny droplets to be used or eliminated by the body, now much of it has to pass directly through the intestinal tract virtually unchanged. Globs of fat in, globs of fat out. You're right, it's gross. That's one reason why, if conditions are addressed early enough, controlling hormone levels might help in the avoidance of surgical intervention.

When the gall bladder does not function properly, the body reacts with an infection. This infection can be so severe that it can kill you. If you ever experience severe pain in the upper center or right part of your abdomen, often accompanied by fever, nausea, a bloated feeling, or jaundice (a yellowish coloring of the skin), don't hesitate to hightail it to your doctor or local emergency room.

22

Estrogen Dominance

Estrogen dominance is a term that has become very familiar to many women over the last 15 years. It was coined by John R. Lee, M.D., author of the *What Your Doctor May Not Tell You About* series of books. The efforts of the late Dr. Lee have been landmark in educating the medical community and the public on the topic of natural hormone replacement therapy, in particular on the subject of estrogen dominance. Estrogen dominance describes a condition where a woman can have deficient, normal, or excessive amounts of the hormone estrogen, but have little or none of the progesterone hormone to balance its effects in the body. This means that even a woman with low estrogen levels can have estrogen dominance symptoms if she doesn't have enough progesterone. This estrogen imbalance can result in an excess of estrogen-related symptoms and conditions.

Because it is possible for diagnostic testing (in the form of blood, saliva, and other tests) for hormonal levels to indicate levels in the "normal range" when a condition of estrogen dominance really exists, it is important to be informed about the nature of this condition. If you have a test of this sort and feel it does not reveal something it should, ask your health care provider! The important thing is to find a provider with whom you can work and who works well with you.

Many of the common causes of estrogen dominance and excess are listed below:

- obesity (estrogen is made in fat cells; excess fat = excess estrogen)
- stress
- poor diet
- nutritional deficiencies
- use of contraceptives
- conventional Hormone Replacement Therapy
- xenohormone exposure (environment- and petroleum-based)
- adrenal fatigue

Many of the common symptoms of estrogen dominance and excess are listed below:

- anxiety, irritability, anger, agitation
- mood swings
- depression
- weight gain
- food cravings (sweets)
- headaches/migraines
- cramps, heavy bleeding
- bloating
- back pain
- acne
- foggy thinking, poor memory
- cold hands and feet
- blood sugar instability

- osteoporosis
- irregular periods
- decreased sex drive
- gall bladder problems
- infertility
- insomnia
- endometriosis
- olycystic ovaries
- uterine fibroids
- cervical dysplasia
- tendency toward developing an autoimmune disorder
- decreased resistance to all forms of cancer
- breast tenderness, lumps, enlargement, and fibrous cysts

23

Progesterone, Testosterone, & DHEA

Making sure that you have a truly correct balance of hormones, something not necessarily evident even when "normal" ranges appear on a lab test, is obviously an important consideration. And there are certainly many great doctors out there who know how to look past the black and white printed numbers on lab test results to see what is really going on and to find out what your body needs. But again, that's why you have to find a physician who is not only right for you but for whom you are right.

Progesterone

A correct balance of hormones is especially relevant with regards to the progesterone hormone, which is produced in the ovaries, adrenal glands, brain, and peripheral nerves. Progesterone is a *steroidal*, or fat-soluble, organic compound with the primary role of balancing estrogen levels. One of the primary functions of progesterone is to prepare the body to sustain pregnancy. Levels of progesterone also typically increase during the second half of the menstrual cycle and contribute to things like food cravings. I know women who, after years of having a monthly cycle, still don't recognize that the cravings they experience are the body's way of telling them that it is trying to prepare the uterus for a possible pregnancy. Instead, they focus on worrying about how eating "too much" for a few days will cause them to gain weight and about how bloated they feel. In reality, regardless of whether or not you give in to the cravings you have, progesterone will continue to do its thing month in and month out. That is why, if your tendency is to be anxious every month that your "unexplained" cravings are going to "make you fat," my advice is to try to relax instead. Your stressing won't keep you from gaining weight (you'll learn why later) or make the cravings go away.

Think of progesterone as the general contractor for your uterus, or womb, where prenatal development occurs. General contractors are responsible for overseeing the building of a structure's walls, roof, and foundation. Progesterone acts in the same way because it is responsible for creating the protective structures, or components, of the uterus. Contractors make sure that electricians and plumbers wire the structure for electricity and gas and provide water and plumbing so that the building will have the elements necessary to sustain its inhabitants. Progesterone helps ensure all the things necessary for a healthy uterus are present and doing their jobs in order to maintain the environment for the development of a healthy fetus.

Progesterone also has a sedative effect to calm you down during times of stress. Can you see how an imbalance of progesterone might cause you to have constant cravings and feel nervous or anxious?

Additionally, progesterone contributes to the body's ability to produce fat. This may come as no big surprise, given what you just learned about how changing progesterone levels can make you feel like eating. But progesterone also slows down how fast the food moves through your gastrointestinal tract. This makes sense because progesterone is providing the body with the time it needs to absorb the nutrients, an important job, especially during the cycle of pregnancy.

This can be a good thing if slowing down means you are absorbing more of a healthy food's nutrients. But progesterone's ability to slow down the progress of food through the system can also have negative ramifications if you are eating a lot of high-fat, simple-carbohydrate foods—typically what many of you eat during times of progesterone imbalance. In those times, you are absorbing more of the very foods that are the opposite of what you—or a potential baby—need most. Furthermore, these are the very foods that get stuck in your system instead of flowing through the way they are supposed to. Additionally, when the body doesn't get the wholesome, natural nutrients it needs, it sends signals to the brain to feed it more. As we've said a number of times, garbage in, garbage out. We could also say, More garbage in, more garbage out—eventually.

The following is a partial list of some of the functions of progesterone:

- helps burn fat for energy
- balances estrogen
- promotes normal cell life cycle
- matures the uterine lining for pregnancy
- contributes to fetal brain and nervous system development
- stimulates bone growth
- helps calm and focus brain activity
- acts as a natural diuretic (increases/maintains normal rate of urination)
- acts as a natural antidepressant
- increases sex drive
- acts as a muscle relaxant
- aids thyroid hormone function
- regulates testosterone
- acts as a preventative of all forms of cancer
- acts as a building block for other steroids

Below is a partial list of symptoms related to progesterone deficiency:

- weight gain
- depression; anger, agitation, irritability
- PMS (Premenstrual Syndrome)
- headaches, migraines
- inability to concentrate; short-term memory impairment
- muscle tension, spasm
- insomnia
- thyroid dysfunction
- fibromyalgia
- osteoporosis
- breast tenderness, lumps, and cysts
- heavy bleeding; clotting; cramping; spotting
- decreased sexual response
- amenorrhea (absent menstrual cycle); oligomenorrhea (infrequent cycles)
- endometriosis (condition where tissue that creates the lining of the uterus can also grow on the outside of the uterus, on the fallopian tubes, ovaries, intestines, and/or other parts of the body, causing pain, cysts, scarring, and/or other complications)
- fibroids
- hot flashes
- water retention; bloating

…and a partial list of symptoms related to progesterone excess:

- sleepiness
- bloating
- constipation

- candida (yeast) infections
- mild depression
- worsened estrogen deficiency symptoms

As I mentioned earlier, progesterone only functions properly when its level is in the right ratio to the body's estrogen level, its primary partner and synergist. Synergy occurs when two or more things work together to achieve more than either one can produce on its own. Remember, Estrogen is necessary to create progesterone receptors and progesterone regulates estrogen receptors. You have to have the right amounts of each.

Progesterone versus progestin

Progesterone, a natural hormone, and progestin, a synthetic hormone, are words that are often used interchangeably in medical literature and research findings. This causes a great deal of confusion, particularly because synthetically manufactured progestins, unlike their natural counterparts, have numerous dangerous side effects, such as breast cancer and birth defects. In 1988 the Federal Scientific Advisory Panel, based on evaluations conducted by the International Agency for the Research on Cancer and by the National Toxicology Program, listed progestins as "a chemical demonstrating evidence of carcinogenicity," in other words, a chemical that causes cancer. Reports about progesterone/progestin may also refer to a symptom or side effect as being "caused by" progesterone, when in fact the symptom or side effect has probably been caused by the progestin in its particular formulation. You'll remember that progestin was the synthetic progesterone given along with the synthetic estrogen (made from horse urine and other chemicals) in the Women's Health Initiative Study and that this study was halted three years early due to a dramatic increase in heart attacks, breast cancer, and cardiovascular disease.

Testosterone: not just for men anymore

Most of us have heard about the hormone testosterone, but only as it relates to men, muscles, and macho. But women have testosterone, too. In women, testosterone is produced in relatively equal amounts in the ovaries and adrenal glands. That's why if a women has a total hysterectomy, where both the uterus and ovaries are removed, has undergone menopause, or experiences any other scenario in which her ovaries slow down or stop functioning, her testosterone (and DHEA) levels can drop to about half their normally produced amounts.

Testosterone levels also contribute to weight regulation. If you're like most women, you've been perplexed and frustrated about the fact that the men you know have always been able to lose weight faster and more easily than you do. Testosterone may well be the reason why. Testosterone is an *anabolic* hormone, which means it helps build muscle and uses fat for fuel. So it won't surprise you to learn that if you had as much testosterone, the powerhouse hormone for building muscle, as men do, you would likely experience the same kind of results. Building muscle is the best way to burn fat because muscle uses fat for fuel more efficiently than any other part of the body. Universal mystery solved! Sorry, ladies. But male or female, ensuring you have the correct levels of testosterone is important for the body's overall balanced functioning.

Possibly one of the greatest benefits of testosterone is that it helps protect the brain against the negative effects of excess cortisol, the hormone produced during times of stress. Research shows that extreme levels of cortisol production can be toxic to brain function and act as a major inflammatory agent. We will discuss cortisol in more detail shortly.

The following is a short list of a few of the many benefits of a correct testosterone level:

- decreased body fat
- lowered cholesterol

- lowered blood pressure
- toned and strong muscle
- bone growth and strength
- increased stamina and energy
- maintained sex drive, or libido
- improved hand-to-eye coordination
- improved wellbeing and mood
- increased blood cell (RBC) production
- decreased insulin resistance
- improved skin health
- improved balance

Dehydroepiandrosterone (DHEA)

Dehydroepiandrosterone, or DHEA, is the most abundant hormone in the blood. DHEA is produced primarily in the adrenal glands, but it can also be produced in the ovaries and brain. Like testosterone, DHEA is an *anabolic* hormone, meaning it helps build body structures.

Very little research was done on DHEA until the mid 1990s. Prior to that time, researchers didn't really understand what it did, but since then research has shown that DHEA plays a major role in cognitive function (thinking and reasoning) and memory. Interestingly, DHEA levels have been shown to diminish with age; this could be one of the reasons for decreased reasoning and memory function in the elderly.

In some preliminary tests, DHEA has shown protective properties against a variety of diseases, including obesity, diabetes, immune disorders, atherosclerosis (the fatty buildup inside of arteries) and cancer. DHEA has been found to:

- increase lean muscle
- play a role in energy, stress, mood and immunity
- thwart cortisol production, resulting in toxicity to the brain and an inflammation

- reverse insulin resistance
- increase strength and stamina
- improve vitality, wellbeing, and vigor
- lower cholesterol, LDLs (the "bad" cholesterol), and triglycerides
- prevent blood clots
- increase bone density
- decrease risk of cardiovascular disease
- increase serotonin levels
- improve the rapid eye movement, or REM, stage of sleep, when sleep is at its deepest
- act as predictor, at lower levels, of heart disease and breast and ovarian cancer
- improve immunity

The fact that DHEA is the primary precursor, or building block, for the body to produce estrogens and testosterone makes it a very important hormone, regardless of how much is actually known about it. Even if that were its only function, however, one would have to say it would be enough.

24

Your Reproductive Organs, What Your Period Is, & Why You Get It

In all probability, the first noticeable "experience" you have had—or will have—with your hormones is due to what is most commonly referred to as your "period" or "menstrual cycle." This chapter provides an overview of the female reproductive system to help you understand exactly why you have a menstrual cycle and what happens when you do.

The anatomy of cycles

You may have also heard this event, called the *ovarian cycle*, described as "that time of the month," your "monthly cycle," your "menses" (the medical term used to describe the first day of the month your flow starts), "menarche" (the onset, or very first time, you experience your flow), or even when your "Aunt Flo (or Bertha or Mary) comes to visit." While the terms for the female reproductive cycle may sound confusing, for simplicity's sake (and you know how much

I love to keep things simple) just know that they are all ways to describe what you probably now think of as "your period," something most girls and women experience on a monthly basis after puberty begins.

A quick, easy-to-understand lesson in anatomy (parts of the body) will be helpful here. As you now know, all the parts of the body you were born with are there for a reason—whether you know/understand the reason or not. In the case of the female reproductive system, or "tract," it's pretty obvious that its reason for being is to reproduce the human species—that is, to make babies.

As in the figure on the next page, the female reproductive organs consist of two ovaries, two fallopian tubes (sometimes referred to as uterine tubes), the uterus, and the vagina. These organs are all located in the lower abdomen area, generally thought of as the area from your belly button down towards the pubic area and between your hipbones. This area might easily be pictured as a broad diamond shape with the belly button at the top of the diamond, the pubic area bones (the bones that lie just under the skin of the vagina) at the bottom of the diamond, and the hips at the sides of the diamond.

The reproductive process starts with something all girls/women produce once they've begun to get their periods: an egg. We are going to follow the path of the egg as it begins in the ovaries and ends, either as part of the flow of your monthly menstrual cycle (your period) or in pregnancy.

> The *ovaries* are glands, called *gonads* (similar in function to the male version of testicles), which are located on each side of the lower part of your abdomen. These two ovaries produce pretty much all of the estrogen and progesterone made in your body and they are also where all your eggs, known as *ova*, are stored.
>
> About once a month an egg leaves the ovaries. The goal of this egg is to travel up into the *fallopian tubes* and then down towards the uterus. This is how it happens:

The Female Reproductive System.

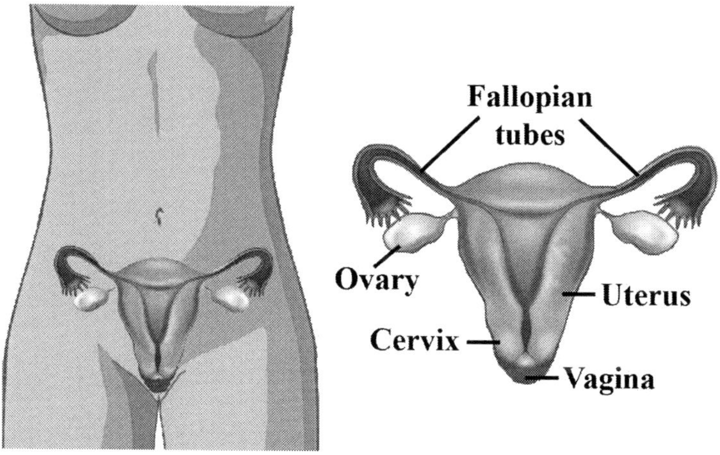

There are two fallopian tubes, each attached to a side of the uterus. The fallopian tubes house tiny passageways no wider than a needle. At the end of the tubes closest to the ovaries are strands of tissue that look something like the end of a mop or fingers. These are called *fimbriae* (pronounced "fim–bree-ee"). The fimbriae's job is to gently direct the progress of the egg when it leaves the ovary by brushing against the ovaries edges. It is this sweeping motion that helps move the egg into the fallopian tube. Once the egg has successfully found its way into the fallopian tube, tiny hairs in the tube's lining help push it down the narrow passageway toward the uterus for implantation or shedding during the period.

The *uterus* is shaped like an upside-down pear, with a thick lining and muscular walls. In fact, the uterus contains some of the strongest muscles in the female body, the kind it takes to expand and contract to accommodate a growing fetus and then help push out a baby during labor. The uterus joins the vagina in the area known as the cervix, which is a shaped like a collar.

At the same time the egg is progressing through the fallopian tube, the lining of the uterus is becoming thicker to make a cushion for a potentially "fertilized" egg. In order for an egg to become fertilized while it is inside the fallopian tube, it must be joined with sperm—the male's version of a reproductive cell or the female egg. If the egg does not join with a sperm cell and does not become fertilized, the lining of the uterus will begin to break down so it can be shed (along with the egg that has not been fertilized). This is when menstrual bleeding begins. In other words, the egg will be passed out of the body as part of the flow of the period. The average cycle of a period takes 28 days to complete. And then it begins all over again.

A note on pregnancy and the uterus

The uterus is positioned comfortably in the lower abdomen. It sits behind the bladder, which helps hold it in place, and in front of the end of the intestinal tract and rectum. Because of the uterus' position, during pregnancy it is common—especially right before the baby is born and sometimes during labor—for the uterus' increasing size to put pressure on both the bladder and the rectum. This makes the woman feel that she has to urinate—even though she may have very little liquid in her bladder.

Inside the uterus

As indicated above, it is the shedding of the uterus' lining (that is, the uterine lining) that causes the bloody flow of menstrual blood each month. More specifically, there are two layers of cells that make up this lining, a thinner *basal* layer and a thicker one, called the *functional* layer. It is this layer that changes so much during menstruation.

Every month the functional layer gets thicker as it fills with blood. It becomes so full that it is referred to as "engorged." This reaction is the body's way of preparing for a fertilized egg. In this case, if a fertilized egg attaches itself to the lining of the uterus it will be able to receive all the nutrients it needs to survive and develop into a fetus—and soon a baby. Again, if there is no fertilized egg to attach to the functional layer, the thick lining full of blood separates from the inner, basal layer and is passed out through the vagina. Because the actual lining itself is released from the uterus and passes out of the body, you may notice darker-colored, long string-like pieces of tissue from the lining that is expelled along with the blood. You may even see small blood clots, or clumps. Bear in mind that all this is part of the normal process of menstruation.

> The *vagina* is a canal-like structure that leads to the uterus and is the connector between the outside of the body and the cervix. It and the cavity of the uterus form the birth canal. The vagina's lining thickens and thins during the menstrual cycle in response to the release of estrogen from the ovaries and is thickest and most elastic during ovulation (the time when eggs are produced) and pregnancy.

Hormones and the reproductive cycle

In terms of hormones, all of your reproductive organs as well as the functions/activities of your menstrual/ovarian cycle are controlled almost entirely by a female's two major hormones, estrogen and progesterone.

The ovaries are the only organs in which large amounts of estrogens are produced; the primary estrogen produced is estradiol. As we know, the hormone estrogen works as a chemical messenger in the body. It is essential for normal sexual development and the functioning of female organs like the ovaries and uterus that are important for childbearing and helps regulate the menstrual cycles. Estrogen is necessary for the normal development of the breasts and helps maintain the heart and healthy bones.

Clearly, estrogens are critical to the body's functioning on many levels. But because estrogens are so powerful, there is also the chance that it may be implicated in the risk for some types of cancer. This is due to its role in stimulating breast cell division, its work during the critical periods of breast growth and development, its effect on other hormones that stimulate breast cell division, and its support of the growth of estrogen-responsive tumors.

[With all this said, however, it's important to recognize that we all have cancerous cells in our body. That's right! We all have cancerous cells, cells that, for whatever reason, have stopped working the way they should and have started to reproduce at a much faster rate than they should, to one degree or another. I share this information with you to give you more confidence in the awesome power of your body. Because when you understand and take care of it, you will be in a much better position to have a healthy, strong immune system, and a strong immune system works to maintain a correct balance of cells in the body.]

The progesterone hormone, primarily produced during the last half of the typical 28-day cycle, is made by the *corpus luteum*, or *collapsed follicle*. We will learn more about the collapsed follicle shortly. In the meantime, it's good to know that progesterone is responsible for the final and critical development of the uterine lining, the lining to which we now know a fertilized egg must attach in order to grow into an embryo. When a pregnancy is successful, progesterone is also the primary hormone responsible for helping support the cells responsible for milk production in the breasts. These are the two major reasons that progesterone is so important during pregnancy. In fact, if progesterone did not do its job effectively, a pregnancy could not occur.

These are just a few more examples of the balance required by your body so it can work like it is intended and you can experience the true health you deserve.

25

Your Eggs, PMS, & Terms You Should Know

What happens after the egg from your mother meets the sperm from your father…but before the person that is you is created?

Conception and after

One of the most significant—and obvious—things that happens during conception is that your gender is decided. This is based on the pairs of chromosomes provided by both your parents. But once your gender is in the bag, so to speak, there are many other characteristics that will begin to be revealed based on that first chromosomal assignment.

One important characteristic that gets decided is that of hormonal makeup. A female's hormones will always be different from a male's, primarily in terms of concentrations, or amounts. This is particularly true for estrogen and progesterone, two hormones that are produced mainly in the ovaries.

Another unique characteristic of being created female is that you are born with all the reproduction cells (eggs) you will ever have! It's true. Unlike males, who continually produce new sperm throughout their lives, you won't make any new eggs at any time in your life because every single egg that may someday be fertilized to reproduce develops with you as part of your original physical package at conception.

According to Arthur Guyton and John Hall, authors of the *Textbook of Medical Physiology* (9th edition), about 8 to 10 weeks before you were born (in the 30th week of pregnancy), "…the number of ova (eggs) reaches about 6 million. Most of [these] soon degenerate, so that only about 2 million are present in the two ovaries at birth and only 300,000 to 400,000 at puberty. Then during all the reproductive years of women, between about 13 and 46 years of age, about 400 of these follicles develop enough to expel their ova (egg)—one each month…." So, though you are born with the number of eggs you will have for your lifetime nestled within your ovaries, they remain relatively under wraps until the onset of puberty, when menstruation begins. What happens then? Your hormones guide and direct your reproduction system to develop and change—to prepare to do what all species do: reproduce. Of course, this does not mean that your hormones have not been hard at work during all those years before you start to notice the changes your physical body is undergoing or before your period actually begins.

On being a girl

From the time you had your very first menstrual cycle (called *menarche*) your reproductive organs as a group understood their role in supporting a fertilized egg (when/if an egg actually becomes fertilized) and in preparing your body for the demands of pregnancy. This means that every single day of every month your hormones are working hard in one capacity or another. There is never a time—ever—when your hormones "take a break" or go on vacation. Which is why if you're not taking care of your hormones the way you should you will probably feel the effects, both physically and emotionally, very quickly.

Generally around age 8 or 9, one part of your brain that starts to work harder is the pituitary gland. The pituitary gland is part of the endocrine system. The goal of the pituitary gland's extra activity is to make more of two specific hormones, FSH (follicle stimulating hormone) and LH (luteinizing hormone). These are the hormones that over the next few years will be responsible for the onset of your monthly period, an event that typically occurs somewhere between age 12 and 16. Of course every girl is different, so the age you will begin or have begun your period will vary depending on many factors. Some of these factors include how well your endocrine, brain, and nervous systems are functioning, how much sleep you get, whether you exercise regularly, what your eating habits are, and the levels of stress in your daily life.

Over the years that your body starts producing more FSH and you get your first period, you will notice a number of significant physical changes. These are called *secondary sexual characteristics* and include breast development, a widening of the hips and waist, and the development of armpit and pubic hair. You may hear a slight change in the pitch of your voice, but typically significantly less than the one boys generally experience. These are all signs your body is helping you take the appropriate steps towards becoming a young woman.

Remember, there are two main "growth activities" that happen during your monthly menstrual cycle. First, the lining of your uterus thickens with blood and nutrients so that if the released egg is fertilized (the start of a pregnancy) it will have the environment necessary for implantation and growth. Second, one of your two ovaries starts producing and releasing one egg at a time. If the egg goes unfertilized, a thickened lining of the uterus will not be required for nutritional purposes. It will therefore be shed, along with fluid and mucus at the time of your menstrual cycle, and leave your body. Your body also uses your monthly cycle as an advantageous way to expel the large amounts of estrogens that are not needed to support a pregnancy. This is an important step in the monthly process because if estrogens are not flushed from the body they can build up and become stored in the body's tissues. Storage of too much estrogen can promote a possibly dangerous, even deadly, situation. Although there are other ways the body detoxifies from potentially trouble-making hormones, this is one of the primary functions of your monthly cycle.

Terminology

Some of the terms related to the female reproductive system might seem like words of a foreign language. If that's the case for you, rest assured that many of the approximately 54 million women between the ages of 14 and 44 (in the United States alone) feel exactly the same way. That's why in this next section I've put together a short glossary of words that I think will be helpful for you to know—and understand. After all, anything that is unfamiliar or confusing can serve to make us uncomfortable or stressed. In the case of hormones, worrying about what we *don't* know only serves to cause more stress—and the hormonal imbalances we are trying to avoid.

The following are very brief definitions of some of the most common terms associated with a woman's monthly cycle.

Puberty: The period of time in a girl's life when secondary sexual characteristics appear, such as the development of breasts, hair growth, primarily in the armpits and pubic area, and a widening and/or a change in the shape of the hips, usually accompanied by additional fat in the hips, thighs, and buttock areas. Puberty usually occurs between age 9 and 13. One of the most noticeable things that happens during puberty is the onset of the first menstrual cycle, or period.

Period/menstrual period / menstrual cycle: The terms most commonly used to describe the time of month during which a woman experiences vaginal bleeding. This normally occurs about every 28 days if the egg released from the ovaries is not fertilized and when the uterine lining is expelled from the body. Generally it is the number of days that a women experiences bleeding that characterizes this period, or cycle.

Menstrual/menstruation: Most often associated with the term *period*, menstruation encompasses the process where the body expels the unfertilized egg, uterine lining, blood, mucus, and fluids over a period of about 2 to 6 days. It is during this "period" that symptoms of cramps, nausea, pain, headaches, irritability, moodiness, insomnia, depression or sadness, anxiety, and/or bloating are most noticeable. These symptoms are often referred to as *premenstrual syndrome*, or PMS.

PMS (premenstrual syndrome): PMS is a "syndrome" characterized by the experience of any combination of the symptoms mentioned above. For most girls and women, such symptoms generally start a few days prior to the onset of the blood flow.

Menses: Blood, fluid, mucus, and tissue of the uterine lining shed that is during the monthly cycle. This is also the medical term used to describe what is most commonly referred to as a "period."

Menarche: The first period a girl has, usually occurring between 9 and 13 years of age. It is not unusual for some girls to experience their first period at age 14 or older.

Menorrhea: A "typical" monthly flow as described above. This term is relatively uncommon, but signifies that "normal" and natural element of getting one's period. You can remember what it means by the "*nor*" in the middle of the word—something you will "normally" experience every month. The discomfort, pain, cramps, nausea, and so on are part of this "normal" process, so don't be concerned if any or all of them occur. If you experience severe or extreme symptoms of any kind, however, never hesitate to consult with your healthcare provider.

Dysmenorrhea: Symptoms such as the ones listed above become "abnormal" when they are severe or extreme. This includes experiencing what you would consider an unusual amount of discomfort or pain, hard cramps that last a long time, extreme nausea, or a much heavier flow than usual. You may have to experience a few monthly cycles before you are able to determine what "typical" symptoms are for you.

Amenorrhea is the absence of a monthly cycle. There are times when not having a monthly period (not bleeding) is completely normal; for example, during the years prior to puberty, the months during pregnancy when the nutrient-rich lining of the uterus is supporting a growing baby, and during the years when a woman transitions into *menopause* when monthly cycles stop altogether.

Girls and women who have low amounts of body fat and/or who are highly athletic may also experience inconsistent periods or periods that stop altogether. This may be due to the fact that since hormones are made from cholesterol, or fat, when the body fat ratio becomes too low, hormone levels may also trend below normal production.

Menopause is the stage of a woman's life when her hormone levels naturally begin to decline as she matures. Ultimately, she will transition to a time where she stops having monthly menstrual cycles. This is typically a gradual process with lighter and less frequent monthly cycles. Typically, menopause can occur anywhere from the mid-30s to the early 60s before the process comes to completion.

Hysterectomy: In some instances menopause is artificially induced when a woman's reproductive organs are surgically removed through surgery called a *hysterectomy*. This is undergone for a variety of medical conditions we won't take time to discuss here. There are different types of hysterectomies, including removal of the uterus alone, removal of both the uterus and the cervix (a total hysterectomy), removal of the uterus, cervix, ovaries, fallopian tubes, and lymph nodes, and radical (complete) hysterectomies (removal of the uterus, cervix, ovaries, fallopian tubes and a portion of the upper vagina), sometimes undertaken in cases of cancer.

It is important to remember that the ovaries are the primary site of estrogen and progesterone production. Therefore, if the ovaries are removed, side effects and symptoms associated with their loss occur. Since these side effects affect hormonal balance throughout the body's system, hormonal supplementation is required to help offset the imbalances. Many patients share with me the fact that they have had their ovaries removed and are not on any type of hormonal supplementation. In these cases, I immediately refer them to a local practitioner who works with bioidentical hormones. With appropriate guidance, these women are often able to relieve—if not completely alleviate—the vast array of symptoms they tend to experience. The most common of these symptoms include weight gain, fatigue and/

or lack of energy, moodiness, and continual feelings of unhappiness.

Choosing not to have a period

While we're on the subject of menorrhea (a normal monthly cycle) and amenorrhea (when there's no monthly cycle), it has been an increasing matter of concern for me that apparently more and more girls and women are currently experiencing what I refer to as "intentional" amenorrhea—the lack of a monthly cycle due to taking birth control pills or injections. These birth control methods are doing what they are supposed to do by keeping the monthly cycle—that is, the possibly of pregnancy—from occurring. My question is, if we're keeping a normal and necessary function of the body from occurring, what other effects might this "abnormal" intervention be having on girls and women everywhere?

I can hear the cry go up, "But you're a guy, you just don't understand what it's like!" And you're right—in the sense that there is no way I can understand what women go through physically, emotionally, or hormonally during their monthly menstruation cycles. On the other hand, I *do* understand pretty darn well how the body works, or is intended to work, and that when humans interfere or intervene with a natural process, there is a high probability a negative outcome will be right around the corner.

Interestingly, most of the women and girls I know say that the reason they start birth control in the first place is not to control pregnancy. In fact, the primary reason given by these individuals is that what they really want to "control" are the monthly symptoms related to their period, symptoms that seem to have gotten out of hand and have become "unbearable."

Trust me, I get the message. But at this point I hope you are beginning to understand that the reason for such symptoms is more about a hormonal imbalance than it is about menstruation itself. And that when hormones are not working the way they should, the inconvenience of having a monthly period can be magnified. Drugs like the pill or birth control injections may seem like an easy fix, but in the long run I fear that the long-term negative impact on the bodies of many, many girls and women will far outweigh any possible benefit they may feel they achieve in the short run.

Furthermore, I believe there are some very basic reasons why so many girls and women are suffering from debilitating symptoms relating to their monthly cycles. These include the usual culprits: poor nutritional/eating habits, a lack of condition-specific nutritional supplements, too little water and WAY too many high-sugar drinks, not enough sleep, and entirely too much stress. Although many helpful suggestions are made for correcting these issues in this book, you can also find additional support on our website, www.hormonebasics.com.

26

Cortisol & Stress & Their Devastating Effects

Of all the hormones we've discussed, cortisol, known as the "stress hormone," may very well be having the greatest effect on your life. That's why it deserves a chapter all its own. I don't like to be harsh, but from personal experience I know that what you don't know about cortisol can literally suck the life out of you. What happens then? You die.

Unless you've been in a cave or stranded on a desert island, you are likely hearing more and more about stress because there is more and more information available about how it is related to most all diseases and dysfunctions of the body. It has been estimated that stress may be an underlying factor in as many as 80 to 90% of all health problems. So, you probably don't need a scientist or doctor to tell you that too much stress is not a good thing, especially when it becomes *dis*-stress. Do you feel you are in a state of distress some—or most—of the time? If you do, you are not alone.

Cortisol, the fight or flight hormone

The state of our stress is controlled by our levels of cortisol, which in turn react to our levels of stress, and so on. *Mosby's Medical Dictionary* defines *cortisol* as a "steroid hormone, also known as a corticosteroid; produced by the adrenal system that influences or controls key processes of the body, including the immune system, inflammatory processes, carbohydrate and protein metabolism, maintenance of serum glucose levels, electrolyte and water balance, and functions of the cardiovascular system, skeletal system, kidneys, and other organs."

Less is known about cortisol than many of the other hormones scientists have studied to date. That's probably why many of us aren't familiar with its qualities. But cortisol is an extremely powerful hormone. In fact, it is a master controller of numerous systems, processes, actions, and organs in the body, so much so that it affects all aspects of health. That's why when cortisol levels are out of whack, everything that cortisol affects will be out of whack, too.

The reason cortisol is known as the "fight or flight" hormone is that its release in the body is due to our reaction to stress—the kind that makes us either want to stand up to and fight or run from whatever stress has presented itself. This doesn't necessarily mean we literally stay to physically fight or physically take flight. It may mean dealing with or avoiding whatever comes our way. It may mean suppressing whatever emotional stress we feel, or choosing to face it in a healthier, more productive way.

Cortisol is the major hormone produced by the adrenal glands in response to any psychological (mental) or physical stressor. We tend to use the word "stressed" to describe when we feel uptight, wound up, anxious, or out of control. We might say that we feel shaky or unable to cope. But according to the dictionary definition of "stress," there are actually three types the body faces: physical, emotional, and chemical.

Physical stress

Physical stress is the kind of stress you feel when you push your body too hard. You don't have to be a lumberjack, marathon runner, or weight-lifter to stress your body physically. In fact, the majority of people who suffer from the physical stress of day-to-day living do so with little to no actual strenuous physical activity. Too little sleep, too many appointments or obligations, sitting too long, standing too long, repeating the same motions over and over again, working in the yard, working at the computer, and even cleaning house are all examples of ways you may be over-stressing your body on a physical level. Our bodies are made to work and function, but not without proper support and care. Staying rested and nourished and paying attention to how we perform certain activities are all part of the big picture in reducing physical stress.

Emotional stress

The next type of stress is emotional. This is the type most people consider the biggest troublemaker. I doubt an in-depth, scientific explanation of emotional stress is necessary here. If you don't know what emotional stress is, you may well be one of the only people on earth living a stress free life. In that case, though, I'd probably say you had to be in complete denial. But if you are like the rest of us who recognize that stress of one kind or another permeates much of our daily lives, you can take your pick as to which particular elements in your life are the cause.

Most of my patients tell me the two primary causes of their emotional stress are money and family. The money issue appears relatively simple: less money means more stress. Frankly, most people feel as if they don't have enough money, regardless of the fact that "enough" is a relative term. But even those people who feel they have plenty of money and therefore aren't stressed about paying their bills admit to feeling stress around the subject of money. It's possible, for example, for people who feel they have more than enough money to feel stressed about the possibility of losing it. You might think that would be a nice problem to have, but either way, if it becomes a source of worry, it will have a negative effect on you and your health.

When it comes to family, well, the sky's the limit. Family relationships, whether with a parent, sibling, grandparent, aunt, uncle, cousin, spouse, kid, or any other family member, have the potential to be mine fields of stress and strain. And because families generally don't go away, neither does the stress they bring with them. None of us are immune to this type of stress. And because our problems are ours, they are always the most important, the biggest, and the worst. The problems of a coworker or a friend are never quite as important to us, simply because they aren't our problems. It's true that some of us also let the problems of others affect us indirectly, even when we are not always conscious that we're doing so. In the end, the degree to which we let other peoples' problems affect us is up to us and us alone.

There are more and more studies showing how emotional stress affects the body and emphasizing the correlation emotional stress has to disease and dysfunction. There are also countless psychology and self-help books that have been written on stress and how to offset it, many of them extremely helpful to those of us who need help. We don't have the space to discuss all those techniques here. Suffice it to say that, according to the results of a 2007 survey by the American Psychological Association, one third of all Americans are living with "extreme stress" and nearly half (48%) believe that their stress has increased over the past five years. Stress is clearly taking a toll on people—contributing to health problems, poor relationships, and lost productivity at work.

As stress in America continues to escalate it affects every aspect of our lives—from work to personal relationships to sleep patterns to eating habits to health. "We know that stress is a fact of life and some stress can have a positive impact," says psychologist Russ Newman, Ph.D., J.D., A.P.A., Executive Director, Professional Practice, American Psychological Association.

"However, the high stress levels that many Americans report experiencing can have long-term health consequences, ranging from fatigue to obesity and heart disease."

You should know that you don't have to believe or even acknowledge that you have stress of any type for it to affect you. You can deal with your stress starting today or you can deal with the affect of the stress and what it creates later, but this is definitely a situation where sooner than later is the best policy.

Chemical stress

The last classification of stress is chemical stress, the type of stress that affects us due to the damage from chemicals on the body. As we've discussed, the list of chemicals that bombard us every second of our lives is pretty much endless and continues from the minute we're born to the day we take our last breath. And those persistent organic pollutants aren't going away any time soon.

I think it's common to think of "chemicals" in relation to scientific experiments or elements of products created by factories—in essence, things we can sort of put in the back of our minds and ignore. Unfortunately, many of these (in fact, most of these) end up in the water we drink, the land where we live, in our homes, our pesticides, our cleaning products, and so on. They're all around us and end up *in* us all the time.

To take any kind of action that fights this bombardment is therefore really important. As I've said, start reading those labels on the things you use everyday: makeup products, such as blush, eyeliner, foundation, lipstick, eye shadow; personal hygiene products, such as toothpaste, deodorant, hair spray, shampoo, conditioner, nail polish, and nail polish remover; gardening products and household cleaners—well, you get the gist. Even the "natural" products will have ingredients that may astound you in their not-so-natural ability to affect the human body in a less-than-positive manner.

In all likelihood you are right now absorbing chemicals from the clothes you are wearing and the laundry soap and fabric softener you used on them. If you are on any medication, prescription or over the counter, it is almost guaranteed that it is having some negative affect on your body, even though it was prescribed to benefit you in some way. I am not telling you to stop taking your medication; you should never self-medicate, stop, or adjust your medication without consulting your health care provider. Just understand that you may not be aware of certain negative aspects outside of the known side effects of the medication you're taking. (Note: If you are one of the millions of Americans who are taking more than two prescriptions, also known as a "chemical cocktail" or "prescription cocktail," I strongly advise you to talk with your pharmacist. Prescription "A" and prescription "B" each has its own set of side effects; when you combine them, it is possible an entirely new list of different side effects, not typically associated with either one, may appear.)

Chemical stress also occurs from the foods we eat. If the majority of what you are eating does not include organically grown fruits and vegetables, lean, natural meat, and so on, you are probably consuming foods riddled with chemicals. You know that chemicals come in the form of additives, preservatives, artificial colorings and flavors, and hormones. You know that chemicals are used for a variety of reasons, reportedly to "improve" taste and preserve freshness, but mostly to increase the amount of time an item can remain unused and still be edible, the period of time known as the item's "shelf life." These are the ones used in the margarine and fast food, the ones that kept the "foods" in our experiments from degrading. So next time when you pick up that item in the store, read the ingredients. Ingredients are listed in the order of how much of each one is in that particular product. It is scary to see that on many of the labels of many products the first ingredient listed is not the product itself!

Because many Americans' diets consist mainly of what comes out of a box, bag, or can, they are eating highly processed foods with minimal, if any, nutritional benefits and maximum amounts of preservatives and chemicals. This daily chemical overload stresses your body and its ability to rid itself of so many toxins. It takes its toll on your detoxifying organs—the liver, kidneys, lungs, intestinal tract, and even the skin—all of which are working overtime to help keep your body as healthy as possible by processing and excreting waste and toxins. If you don't get rid of these toxins, there is simply nowhere for them to go. Instead, they simply build up inside you, creating a vehicle for a walking, talking waste dump.

Minimizing stress

It is vital to your health to minimize stress, whether it comes from physical, emotional, and/or chemical sources. While it may seem overwhelming—and stressful!—to figure out where to start to reduce your stress, I always suggest keeping it simple and taking one step at a time. You will never escape all sources of stress, so keep it in perspective and remember that worrying doesn't really change anything—other than making you more worried and more stressed, which naturally defeats the purpose. Higher levels of stress then make your stress hormone, or cortisol, level skyrocket as well. In fact, the release of cortisol can increase to as much as 20 times during stressful situations, especially stress that is a result of anxiety or severe injury. This can be a vicious, no-win cycle.

With obligations from work or school and family, we as a society seem consumed by stress. We set our alarm clocks to wake up early enough to try to get everything done even though we know at the end of the day we will still have a full list of things to do that are waiting for us the next day, creating a never-ending onslaught of commitments and responsibilities. The truth is that for the most part we have forgotten how to control the various aspects of our lives or, more importantly, that we *can* control them.

But you can change the outlook of your life—should you choose to change it. Like taking the time to read this book. Making yourself a priority and taking care of yourself is imperative to your physical and mental wellbeing. I often tell my patients that if they don't take care of themselves, they may not be able to take care of anyone else. The truth is that I've seen this play out time and time again.

Worrying

It's important to understand that no one else is the cause of your stress, because ultimately you are the one in control. If you do not allow yourself to feel stressed, you won't be stressed. Of course it's never quite that simple in life, but recognizing the truth behind this statement helps. Remember: no one else has the means to cause you to be stressed! The nature of stress is that it erases the potential for a positive outcome, whether for you, someone else, or the situation. My advice, the advice I often give myself and try to take, is to lighten up and to focus on the positive, not the negative.

If you find yourself worrying constantly about paying bills, making good grades, who likes or who doesn't like you, or about finding a job, all you are doing is making yourself miserable. Unless you can find a job and get paid to be a worrier, you are getting absolutely nothing positive accomplished. If there were a company that paid people to worry, no one would go jobless, right? Admittedly, with the economy in such tough shape, we could all wake up and go to sleep in the same anxious state. But beginning and ending your day in a stressful state only keeps the negative cycle going.

Possibly you are worried about your friends, significant other, kids, or family members. There are plenty of reasons to worry, if that's what you choose to do. What if your parents become ill or are unable to take care of themselves? What if your kids don't do well in school or start running with the wrong crowd? What if the unthinkable happens and they come to harm? What if someone you love is in an accident or gets sick?

Is this how you spend your day…or even a part of it? If you stop worrying for only a minute to clear your head and heart you may want to think about this: you can never worry enough to make someone like you or love you. You can never worry enough to keep someone well or safe, to stay young, to be smart, or anything else.

All worrying does is make you worry more. Furthermore, worrying makes you sick. Literally. Unless you believe you are God or some other entity controlling what happens in life, worrying wastes positive energy units. And in my estimation most of us aren't supreme beings, even though we may expect ourselves to have that kind of power. So *quit worrying*.

And please don't fool yourself into thinking, "Oh, but I don't worry about bad things happening. I only think about wanting good things to happen." While I believe you probably *do* want only the good things to happen, how you think, speak, and feel about it may tell a different story.

Here's an example. If some type of illness or disease runs in your family and you spend time thinking, "I expect NOT to get what other family members have had and I expect my kids WON'T get what they had," that's negative thinking. You aren't wishing *for* good health or attracting health into your life with this kind of language. Using "not," a negative word, is self-defeating. "Don't" is negative. "Do" is positive. Think, speak, and live what you DO want. A way to re-think, re-speak, and re-feel this would be: "I love how healthy I am and how healthy my family is; we will continue to be well and happy because we eat well, exercise, get plenty of sleep, and do all the things we can to stay that way."

Your heart and soul's intent may be the same, but sometimes we allow the message to become convoluted. When you stay positive, in part by expressing what it is you really want, you should notice immediately that your stress levels go down in direct correlation. Your distress may even disappear. Many people report that good things start to happen to them and to others around them when they let go of their negative thinking patterns. In essence, they have opened the door to a life without the negative effects of too much stress.

Because things are going to happen and people are going to do what they do regardless of how much you stress or worry, it helps to stop putting so much pressure on yourself by assuming you have the power to control those things you don't.

It is my belief that we only have so many positive energy units in a day and when they are gone we stop being a productive, positive influence on our environment. If we run out of positive energy, all we have left is negative energy, or neutral energy at best. If our energy hovers around neutral long enough, the trend often gravitates towards the negative. We end up running on empty, the way too many people are living their lives. Anxiety does more to your body and mind than cause fatigue, irritability, sleeplessness, wrinkles, stomach issues, acne, and headaches. That's just the tip of the iceberg. Stress and its chemical by-products may be setting you up for more life-threatening conditions.

George P. Chrousos, M.D., a prominent clinical investigator in the field of stress, says, "The body's response to stress can be harmful as well as helpful. The same mechanism that commands alertness and focus in tense situations may eventually harm the body if constantly triggered." Dr. Chrousos goes on to explain that "More than 25% of American adults have stress-related metabolic syndrome, which is the most common cause of death in the Western world." The major components of metabolic syndrome are abdominal obesity, dyslipidemia (high cholesterol), high blood pressure, and blood sugar intolerance, which leads to Type 2 diabetes.

The variety and severity of health problems of people with chronically high levels of cortisol may shorten their life expectancy by 15 to 20 years if left untreated. For some stress-related disorders, women are at a greater disadvantage than men because estrogen stimulates the production of CRH, or the corticotropin-releasing hormone, which can elevate cortisol levels. So women in particular need to get their stress under control. *Please.*

27

Run-in with Reality

I personally have learned the hard way how stress can affect every aspect of a person's life. In fact, I'd go so far as to say that I could be a poster child for how ignoring chronic stress can lead to a debilitating illness—or death. I'm going to share my story here so you might learn from my mistakes.

My story is about how "little" signs and symptoms that something is wrong eventually get bigger, and how they finally get so much bigger that you can't ignore them anymore. As I've said before, men have hormones too, but in very different amounts from women. This means that as a woman your overall experience may be dramatically more serious than mine was. Still, the confusion, discomfort, and fear I felt could rival anyone's.

My personal experience started in the way it probably starts for many people—with high levels of stress. I know now that this extreme stress caused a severe cortisol imbalance in my body and that cortisol is the "fight or flight" hormone. I had chosen to live with the stress in my life instead of changing it for a long, long time. When this critical time came to pass at this particular juncture in my life, I was left with no other option than to stay and fight.

I was 32 when I left corporate America to return to school. I had been living in Oklahoma City with my daughter Alex and her mom, but we would soon move to Kansas City when I made the decision to attend Cleveland Chiropractic College.

Alex was 2, going on 3, at the time; her mom was a schoolteacher and coach. Soon I was working 34 to 40 hours a week at a financial services company and attending chiropractic school full-time. Needless to say, my daily schedule was completely full with school, work, studying, and being a husband and a dad. Things were not holding together well and it was during this time that Alex's mom and I decided to divorce. If I hadn't had enough stress already, this put me way over the top, even though I didn't realize it at the time.

I moved out of the small two-bedroom house where we lived and for the next trimester I bounced between classmates and friends who were loving and gracious enough to take me in until I could figure out how to "start over." I made time to see Alex at least every Tuesday and Thursday and every other weekend. Spending time with Alex was the only thing that seemed to keep me going, and not living under the same roof with her was the one thing that continued to tear me apart from the inside out.

The very first time I dropped Alex off after our time together, I cried. To say I bawled would actually be a better description. It was almost a year before I could walk from the front door to the truck after watching her go back into what was once "our" house without the world becoming a blur and without soaking my sleeve with tears. Each time I stumbled blindly through the yard towards the street; once I got inside my truck it was another 20 or so minutes before I could get my crying under control and be capable of driving home. More often than not I had to make frequent stops, sometimes as close as the stop sign a half block up the street, where I cried like a baby. It was either stop the truck or risk a head-on collision. It was like driving in a torrential downpour without windshield wipers.

I refused to cry in front of Alex and it wouldn't have been fair to force my emotional state on whichever friend I was staying with at the time. Even as I began to understand the physiology of how the body worked, I couldn't for the life of me figure out how it could produce so many tears out of just two eyes. But I knew the tears were coming from a dark place deep inside me, a place I had never known existed before.

This trend continued until Alex was almost 6. That's when the crying finally began to taper off. I'm really not sure the pain of that time is entirely gone, however, even today. Not being with my daughter was like having a part of me go missing. My heart physically hurt to the degree where I was afraid I would never recover.

Unless you're crying tears of happiness, tears are generally the result of some sort of stress, usually emotionally induced. Yes, when you cut onions the chemical reaction will make you shed a few tears even if you're happy, but I think you know what I mean. What I've realized over the years is that though the majority of my tears were an emotional reaction to having to live separately from my daughter, there were many other contributing factors involved as well. I was 34ish, a full-time student working a full-time job, with a daughter I missed all the time and was determined to see as much as I could. My plate was full to say the least, but whose wasn't? That's what I kept telling myself.

It was springtime when I first noticed my problem. I was well into school and entrenched in all of the classes on microbiology, cell biology, physiology, neuroanatomy, gross anatomy, and so on. You don't have to be in chiropractic or medical school to know when your body isn't working the way it should—that is, if you just listen to what it's telling you. But I must have had earplugs in, headphones on, a blanket wrapped around my head, and my head buried in the sand. The warnings were there, but for some reason I didn't listen to my body, which was screaming at me that there was a problem and that if I didn't deal with the problem it was going to quit knocking on my door and kick it in.

Anyway, I awoke one spring morning at 7:30. I could feel my heart and pulse pounding, not just in my chest, but also in my head and throughout my entire body. I immediately checked my pulse to find my heart rate was 126 beats per minute. It is important to note two things here. One is that before I had done anything more than open my eyes, I had the wherewithal to check my pulse, so I knew the reading was as true a "resting" heart rate as you could get; and two, for someone my age and in pretty good shape, an average heart rate should have been around 65 beats per minute. This meant it was almost double what it should have been.

At the time I wasn't sure why I wasn't more alarmed than I was. I guess I figured that with everything I had going on my high pulse rate was due to stress and that it would pass as I got my stress under control. Sounds easy, right? But what an unbelievable, crazy, terrifying journey I was about to undertake to make that happen.

A year went by. My heart rate and pulse continued its roller coaster ride from dramatic highs to bottomed-out lows for the entire 12 months. All the while I kept thinking, "I'll get this under control, it's almost over, then I'll be able to calm down and be okay."

Then the time for my national boards came around. Chiropractic students, like medical students, have to sit for national board exams before they can take the state boards for licensure. The first three of the four national boards are comprehensive and consist of 200 questions each. They seem almost impossible to pass. So, if you weren't stressed enough already, with all the assignments and exams in school, getting ready for the national boards would definitely do it for you.

My stress levels catapulted to new heights with every set of boards that I took. Finally, I recognized I needed some kind of a break. Two of my closest friends, Pat and Courtenay, who had met and married while in chiropractic school and were currently in the process of opening a clinic in Austin, Texas, invited me down for a visit and I accepted. We always had a great time together and it was exactly what I needed to begin "de-stressing."

One minor thing I need to mention before I continue. Somewhere along the road to Stressville, my body decided that one way it would deal with stress when things got too crazy was to empty its stomach contents. I don't mean minor league spit-up either. When the stress got too high my body reacted by convulsing. My whole body arched, every muscle went taut, and then spasmed. Every muscle went as tight as a steel cable. The spasms made each of my 10 toes curl in an attempt to empty whatever was in my stomach—if there was anything there to empty. Whether I ate or not, this routine repeated itself over and over and the more stressed I became the more frequently it manifested. If you've ever had the flu and experienced dry heaves, you have some idea what I was experiencing.

My body was under such pressure during these times that my eyes turned black. Usually this occurred only in my eyelids so it often went unnoticed (at least by others), except when the vessels inside my eyes ruptured. My excuse when questioned was that I had coughed too hard. Not a complete lie, but a lie nonetheless. And, as we all know, lies only get you into trouble.

Anyway, this particular weekend I ended up in Austin, one my favorite places to visit, to hang out with two of my dearest friends. The weekend weather was beautiful. Other than a brief early-morning shower the first morning, it was sunny and warm. As we had done many times before, we set off on an adventure, this time south to the town of Gruene, Texas for a concert and some relaxation.

It's interesting how you can convince yourself you're doing something positive for yourself, like taking time away to de-stress, only to find out when you start to unwind that you're coming completely unwound. That's exactly what happened to me. Everything that had been bubbling under the surface came to a raging boil just when I thought my life was about to cool off. My brain had been tricking itself (and the rest of my body) by functioning in a relatively normal state, while my body had been freaking out—operating, but just barely hanging on. Any communication between the two—my brain and my body—was poor at best.

The trip to Gruene and the concert were great, but it was on that beautiful afternoon in south Texas that I emotionally snapped and my meltdown started. I believe the old saying goes, "When you least expect it, expect it." After we got back to Austin, the mother of all dry heaves began. It was so bad that my friend Patrick, who is absolutely a man's man—a born and bred tobacco-chewing Texan who grew up riding motor-cross and hunting anything he could with every type of weapon known to man, and with so much camo it covered part of his truck—knocked on the door of the bathroom and, if I remember correctly, actually came into the bathroom to make sure I was okay. That may not sound like much to you, but when it came to Patrick it was downright warm and fuzzy. I did my best to assure Patrick I was okay and that it would be over soon, but I knew he didn't believe me. Honestly, I didn't believe it myself. I don't know exactly how long I spent in that tiny tiled room, but I do know it was the most violent episode of vomiting and dry heaving I've ever had.

Once the episode was over, I felt lucky that it was just a few short steps to the bed in the spare room where I was staying because not only were my toes curled and cramping, both my feet were cramping also. All I remember before I passed out from exhaustion was that this had to stop. I knew my body and mind couldn't take much more.

The next morning as I opened my eyes I immediately remembered what had happened the previous day and night and felt instant relief that the events were behind me. And that's the moment—that big *ah-hah* that people talk about—when I became starkly aware that I had bigger problems than the incident of less than twelve hours before. Something was not right.

I checked my pulse. It was nowhere near normal and that neither was my heartbeat, a far more serious situation. Most of you know that the heart should beat at a regular, steady interval, even if it's fast, as when you are excited or scared. I hadn't been scared when I woke up, but now I was terrified. I checked my pulse, then again. I couldn't get a steady pulse.

We'd been taught about irregular pulses and heartbeats in school and how to detect them, but it's a whole different scenario when it is happening to you. I checked my pulse over and over, what must have been ten times. The steady, regular beat just wasn't there; the high rate was.

I immediately got up and went downstairs where Patrick and Courtenay were making breakfast. I quickly brought them up to speed on the events of the morning, at which point Courtenay went for her stethoscope while Patrick verified my findings.

I'll never forget the look on Courtenay's face as she shared with Patrick what I already knew. My heart was not only beating a mile a minute, it was out of rhythm. My friends called a Texas trooper friend of theirs who sometimes worked at one of the local hospitals in his off hours. The trooper advised them what I suspect we all already knew: that it was time to get me to a hospital.

It was a slightly cool, incredibly calm, clear Sunday morning as we made our way to the Heart Hospital of Austin in Patrick's tricked-out hunting Suburban. I felt surprisingly calm at first, having experienced many good times in that very Suburban, but it didn't take long before the fear took over. The closer we got to the hospital the more nervous I became. As we all know, when you get nervous your heart beats faster. And that's what happened. My heart beat faster and faster, continuing its out-of-rhythm *ba-boom, ba-ba-boom* the whole time. The unsettling sensations made things worse.

By the time I made it to the reception window in the emergency room, I was having trouble talking and couldn't catch my breath. The nurse was well into her usual shpiel on paperwork, how to fill it out, insurance cards, blah, blah, blah, when she evidently picked up on the word "heart." That's when all the formalities stopped and I was advised to proceed directly through the two stainless-steel swinging doors just to my right. No sooner had the doors swung inward than I was approached by two nurses headed directly for me with a purposeful, rapid pace. Each one took me by an arm and politely escorted me into the first available room. They helped me into bed and hooked me up to a monitor, took my vitals, and proceeded with the usual intake procedures. About the time the nurse on my right got the monitor hooked up and turned on, the alarm went off.

Both nurses looked towards the monitor and then at me, then directly at each other in a way that left no one confused about what was happening. Without a word, the nurse to my left and closest to the door rushed out, while the nurse on my right told me to "calm down." I think she'd said it twice before the door flew open and the medical circus came to town.

In addition to the nurse who had left the room just moments before, three other nurses entered, pushing two carts, making the total nurse count five. Two doctors and a crash cart entered a second later. Crash carts are the carts they wheel in to shock people back to life on television. Turns out they're the same in real life, but this time the scene from television was my life and I was the star.

I knew right then and there this had gone way too far. I was horrified, frozen with fear and panic. They told me to calm down over and over, that "being excited" wasn't helping. *Seriously*, I thought, *I am anything but excited. You try to calm down while…*

Oh, my God, what was that? "That" was the first of two anti-coagulant shots that had suddenly pierced my stomach. As soon as I felt the first needle being pulled from my gut I felt the second go in. It wasn't any better the second time around. Shots in the stomach are an interesting sensation. I don't recommend them.

The doctor to my right was questioning me to try to figure out what had landed me in this condition. He continued to assume it was drugs, alcohol, or a combination. In fact, he refused to acknowledge it could be anything else. I assured him I didn't take drugs of any kind and that the beer I'd had earlier in the evening the day before shouldn't have anything to do with what was now happening. I was busy trying to explain to him something he should already have known.

Time out here for a little doctor-talk.

The tenth cranial nerve is called the *vagus* nerve. It is the only nerve that runs from the brain, through the neck, and into the abdomen. It has many branches off the main nerve, one of which innervates (communicates energy to) the heart, and another, which is associated with the gag reflex. Hence the connection between violent dry heaves and their effect on heart rate and rhythm.

Unfortunately, this ER doc was unwilling to consider the obvious. And what did I know? I was only a chiropractic student whose professional focus was the nervous system. (Read with sarcasm.) The discussion continued in a repetitive cycle. The doctor kept trying to convince me that my problem was due to drugs and I kept trying to explain anatomy to him. At one point in the harrowing ordeal I begged him to do a blood test for drugs as he'd never ordered one. As our cozy little conversation occurred, literal pandemonium was all around us.

At the same time the doctor was interrogating me, he was also instructing the nurse to his left and directly to the right of my head to "turn the monitor higher." As I did my best to answer his questions, he continued to instruct the nurse to turn the monitor higher. I can only assume he was becoming as annoyed as I was with the continual alarm bell that was sounding over and over in a very loud, impossible-to-ignore tone to indicate that my heart rate was dangerously high. It was as if we were right in the middle of the midway at the state fair with all the bells and whistles going off, but there were no foot-long corn dogs, funnel cakes, or prizes to be won.

After about the umpteenth time the alarm went off again, at which time the doctor snapped at the nurse one last time to "turn that damn thing off!" to which she responded frantically, in a pitch and at a level just short of a scream, "It's as high as it will go!"

The suspense finally got the best of me and I turned my head to see what all the fuss was about. Remember when I told you that an average heart rate for someone my age (at that time) would be around 65? Well, the number on the heart rate monitor was 196. I was at least three times over the normal heart rate speed and, because I am a lifetime over-achiever, it was out of rhythm as well.

That was when I lost it. I realized the tears I'd cried for so many months whenever I left Alex at the door were nothing compared to the emotions I felt when I thought about dying, because dying meant I would never see her again.

I had treasured every second of every minute I had ever been able to spend with my daughter and it hadn't been enough. I remembered the night Alex was born. When they put her in my arms all I could do was look at her and cry. I remembered all the times her beautiful little face lit up when I got home. I remembered all the times after the divorce when she looked me right in the eye and asked me, "Daddy, when are you coming home?" I remembered everything about everything that pertained to Alex as I was being forced to come to terms with the fact that it might all be ending as I lay in a hospital bed among strangers. I never felt farther away from those I loved than I did at that moment. I had been the best dad I knew how to be under the circumstances, but I felt as if I had cheated her. She deserved more. She didn't deserve to have to live without a daddy because of divorce and she absolutely didn't deserve to live without a daddy forever because he couldn't get control of his life and his stress.

Oddly enough, in the middle of the alarms going off, tears once again blurring my world and streaming down my face, doctors and nurses shouting at each other and massive confusion, a song popped into my head that was very popular at the time. I think it was number one on the country charts and was called *One More Day* by Diamond Rio. The words were probably meant to be from a man expressing his love for a woman, but at that moment they rang true for me as I thought of my little Alex. All I wanted was "one more day," because then I could tell her all the things I wanted and needed her to know if I could just have one more day. And that's when I made the decision that what happened from that point on was really up to me—and God. I suddenly knew with certainty that I was the one ultimately responsible for ending up where I was, so I was the one that would have to find the way out. And immediately I knew that I would.

Things settled down little by little after that and one by one the nurses and doctors left the room. They had succeeded at stabilizing me, the primary goal for the moment. I spent the biggest part of that

Sunday in the emergency room watching the monitors continue to show me my screwed-up numbers. I kept thinking how the numbers were a direct reflection of the state my life was in at that moment. Completely screwed up.

It was late in the afternoon when something happened that actually made me laugh out loud and it was at that point I knew God was letting me in on a little secret: that I had been living too hard a life, that it was out of control and I needed to slow down.

A nurse I hadn't seen before (and at that point I thought I had seen just about all of them) popped her head in the door. She wasn't there to take my vital signs, get me a blanket, pour me water, or anything else. She was there to ask a question.

"So," she asked, "did you win?"

"What?" I was dumbfounded. *What was she talking about?*

"Did you win?" she asked again.

"Did I win what?" I asked. I knew I'd heard correctly, so I waited, unsure, wondering where she was going with this.

"The Austin marathon was today. After I heard how high your heart rate was and what happened to you, I figured you must have run in the race. So, did you win?"

Instinctively I laughed. It felt great. It was then I knew I was going to be okay and that God had a sense of humor. My advice? Remember to acknowledge God's little messages—whether you understand them at the time or not. Because it has been my experience that if God's little taps on your door to get your attention go ignored, He may choose to kick your door in next time around.

I spent the next two days in the Heart Hospital on intravenous medication that would hopefully reset my heart rhythm. The concern with an out-of-rhythm heart is the development of blood clots, which can kill you immediately. Blood clots can form in a very short time, so once you know your heart isn't beating correctly treatment is imperative. I was in what's called *atrial fibrillation*, or "a-fib," as the medical professionals say.

The two top chambers of my heart were fluttering more than pumping; that allowed blood to pool in my heart. Because the doctors estimated that I had probably been in a-fib since the night before, after my dry-heaving episode over twelve hours earlier, it was absolutely a blessing from God that no clots had formed. I received many blessings, some of which I would only fully realize in the days, months, and years to follow. In fact, the entire episode was a blessing, even though you can be sure I didn't see it that way at the time.

I continued to focus all my attention on having my heart revert to its normal rhythm while on the medication, because if it didn't when Tuesday rolled around they were going to have to reset it the old-fashioned way—by shocking it. The fear around that possibility evidently convinced my body to find its way home, because early that Tuesday morning my heart reverted to a normal rhythm and I was released the next day with orders to follow up with a cardiologist as soon as I got back to Kansas City.

I was actually given a great many directives and suggestions, but none of them made mention of how completely fatigued and sore my body would be. I imagine anyone who has had the misfortune of having a heart attack has experienced a similar response and knows just how uncomfortable it is.

I slept the entire trip home. I couldn't walk more than five or six steps before I needed to stop to catch my breath. I know it sounds crazy, but it's true. My conversations became limited to what I could say while exhaling, as I couldn't breathe and talk at the same time. It was impossible and too exhausting. I slept more than I was awake. I felt as if I were in my 90s (with no offense to those who are).

I was told when I left the hospital in Austin that if I experienced any chest pain or went into a-fib again to get to the local emergency room immediately. Unfortunately, two nights after I got home I started having pain in my chest so I did what I had been told. In the local ER, I finally found a doctor who listened to all the events that had led up to my BIG EXPERIENCE and agreed with me that it was undoubtedly the vagus nerve that in all likelihood was causing my problem. Additionally, this doctor told me that part of the reason I was so worn out and sluggish was due to the beta-blockers I had been prescribed to keep my heart and system slowed down. "Those are for people who are much, much older," he said. "No wonder you feel so lousy. You don't need them anymore. But it does sound like you need to get your stress under control."

Hmmm. Exactly.

My pain that night turned out to be nothing more than another one of God's little ways of putting me in touch with someone in the mainstream medical community who would level with me on what was really going on and what I needed, even though I believed I already knew what that was. I don't remember that doctor's name, but I am grateful to him.

After a thorough checkup with the cardiologist, including blood work and a stress test, I was given the same bit of helpful advice. "There is absolutely nothing wrong with your heart and no damage was done. Get your stress under control or you may not get another opportunity," he said. Kudos to him for recommending I see a psychologist—or do whatever it would take to manage my stress—and that's exactly what I did.

It took me almost six weeks before I was able to carry on a normal conversation or do anything without instant fatigue. It was six months before I was pretty much back to normal. No one ever did a test to figure out how much stress (cortisol) was really involved in this equation, but it doesn't take a rocket surgeon to figure it out. (Rocket scientist...brain surgeon...get it?)

Cortisol, stress, animals, and the human body

Looking back to that time, I wonder if I had known what I know today, would I have done things differently? Would I have made more of an effort to set things right in my life before the physical and emotional stress and pain took such a toll? I like to think so. But I do know that when your cortisol levels increase, the major systems of your body are put on a temporary hold. Functions like digestion, growth, reproduction, and the immune system slow down, become almost secondary in the way they behave. That's why chronic stress increases your chances of getting sick, can increase stomach and intestinal problems and often results in skin conditions like acne, hives, rashes, and flushed cheeks. With your mind and body in what is essentially a state of metabolic overdrive, you are always "prepared" to respond to a life-threatening situation. Even when none really exists.

Abnormal levels of stress result in abnormal amounts of cortisol in the body. Elevated cortisol levels can decrease the digestive processes by 50%. Slowing down the digestive process can slow down the body's motility function. Motility is the action your intestinal tract performs to move food through the system to be absorbed and eventually excreted.

We've talked about what happens when the system of excreting toxins malfunctions or doesn't perform as it should. Could this lack of functioning keep the body storing more than it should? Could it be contributing to the obesity epidemic we are experiencing?

If you are wondering why so many major bodily functions are affected by cortisol, the answer may be one based on what we call the survival instinct. A long time ago, as far back as prehistoric times, we lived as hunters and gatherers. Eventually, we, that is human beings, realized we were more likely to survive if we banded together in groups. Because we could not go to the local drive-through when we were hungry, we had to pick up the weapons we had made and hunt for food. While we had no food charts, doctors, or experts to tell us what we should eat and in what quantities, our bodies inherently knew what they needed. Since we were herbivores and/or carnivores, our diets consisted of vegetables, grains, seeds, berries, and often the meat of other species.

One of the major problems with hunting is that a hunter can quickly become the hunted. While stalking one animal he can be pursued himself, perhaps by a saber-toothed tiger or some other carnivorous beast also in need of a protein fix. When face to face with inherent danger, the human entrée-to-be has one of two choices: panic, freeze, and surely become dinner, or react with every instinct available to escape impending doom.

This is where cortisol came in handy for our ancestors. The release of cortisol into the bloodstream allowed for the dramatic reduction of certain functions of the body that required great amounts of energy so that the needed energy could be used in a more productive way at that moment—like figuring out a way to avoid ending up a large carnivore's next meal. How does this happen? Blood flow to the extremities decreases; pupils dilate so the brain can gather more light as well as information; the stomach and intestinal functions grind to a screeching halt; chemicals to "excite" the entire physical system flood the body and senses and tell us to vacate the area as soon as possible, while we're still in one piece. What is this way of dealing with a stressful situation? The fight or flight option: choose to flee or choose to stay.

These responses are the same natural bodily responses that have been occurring since humans have existed in the world. The difference is that the saber-toothed tiger of today might be a narrowly avoided car wreck, news that a loved one is in the hospital or you've just been laid off, having a pop quiz sprung on you at school when you haven't studied, seeing your child fall off of the swing, watching your pet run into the road in front of oncoming traffic… or any one of a million other scenarios that frighten, startle, or excite your system. Because all of these set off an exponential number of chemical, emotional, and physical reactions in your body.

Think about the last time you were driving in your car and about to shift lanes. Think about how you shifted your eyes from the road to insert another CD into the player. Do you remember how you felt the moment when you heard the blaring of the horn from the car that was suddenly directly beside you? In reality, all the sensations you felt in these circumstances were only a fraction of the reactions occurring inside the body that were making it possible for you to respond accordingly by swerving away quickly to avoid a collision—in other words, making it possible for you to choose "fight" or flight, the only available options.

Animals are a great example. Consider zebras. Zebras in the wild have distinct times during their day when they go into the fight-

or-flight mode, compared to other times when they pretty much just hang out, eat, and look for water. During those times when they are concerned for their safety, perhaps pursued by lions or cheetahs, the zebras' chemical levels go through the roof. The interesting thing about the zebras is that as soon as the threat of danger is over (if they are still alive, that is), within moments their bodies automatically revert to the same calm state they were experiencing while they were grazing a few short moments prior. This is because Zebras have systems that allow them to go from 0 to 60 and back to 0 again about as fast as they got there. This is explained in detail in the book *Why Zebras Don't Get Ulcers*, by biologist and Stanford University neuroscientist Robert Sapolsky. Sapolsky explores why zebras don't get heart disease, diabetes, or other chronic diseases the way humans do and how this information relates to stress.

Briefly, unlike the zebras, whose systems go from 0 to 60 and then back to 0 again so quickly, humans find themselves unable to respond the same way. Although we too go from 0 to 60 quickly, we are unable to naturally return to point 0 as quickly. Sometimes we can't get back to point 0 at all. If a high level of continuous stress in our lives makes it impossible to return to what might be a "normal" state of calm, we stay at a level somewhere around 30 or 40 and operate from that level all the time. This continual heightened state of stress becomes the new baseline and sets us up for many of the health problems we end up experiencing.

With every new occurrence of a stressor, your level rises even more, until you eventually blow right past 60 and keep going. This means your baseline goes higher and higher also. You should know enough now to see how detrimental this is to your health! And so, unlike zebras, that never have weight problems, heart disease, cholesterol issues, mental issues, or acne—and that need to stay healthy or give up their lives to the lion or tiger—we are in trouble. Many of our health issues, and all of the potential side effects of these health issues, are due to chronic, excessive stress. As such, they are now major health concerns that lead to a number of life-threatening conditions.

28

Stress & Your Immune System

When I was growing up, the term "immune system" conjured up thoughts of a mystical, ghost-like fog that moved around in my body while it looked for ways to kill the bad stuff that could hurt me or make me sick. I now know the immune system is much more than a fog, but it still remains downright mystical in its phenomenal ability to defend us against the millions of bacteria, microbes, viruses, toxins, and parasites that are either inside our bodies or waiting for the opportunity to invade our bodies. An intricate network, the immune system includes the *thymus*, *spleen*, *lymph nodes*, *macrophages*, *lymphocytes*, and *antibodies*. Fortunately, you don't have to understand what these things are to put them to work for you.

Stress and the immune system

One of the things that most affects the immune system's ability to stave off disease is—you guessed it—stress. Stress is underrated and often ignored in its role as one of the most powerful agents in undermining the immune system's capabilities.

The lymph system is one component of the immune system. One of the jobs of lymph fluid is to absorb and carry away the proteins and waste products produced by the cells, as well as to detect and remove any bacteria that finds its way into the body. You may have already heard about lymph nodes because they are often associated with being sick. When you go for a physical, normally the doctor will check the lymph nodes under your jawbone and in your neck for a sign of illness. This is because when the lymph nodes are swollen or tender, it often means that the lymphs are doing their job—in other words, attempting to collect and eradicate the bacteria, toxins, and so on that may have moved in and made themselves at home.

In the September-October 2001 issue of *Psychophysiology*, Ohio State University researchers reported that stress from engaging in a memory task activates the immune system, whereas stress that results from passively watching a violent video weakens the immune system. These results suggest that deadlines and challenges at work, school, or home, if limited in duration and intensity, can actively and effectively strengthen the body's defenses. The difference is in the type of stress, whether it is positive and productive, such as when you're readying for a competition or getting married, or negative, such as when you have a prolonged argument with a relative. Unfortunately, the reality is that most of us are way past the point of having only a "little" stress (remember the zebras) and of having mostly "positive" stress. As shown in the study, the type of stress you are experience can play a big role in how your body responds over time.

External stressors

Violence is one of those negative stressors. If we stop to think for a moment about how much violence we see on a daily basis—from video games to the news, it's almost impossible to avoid—we can see that it may be having a considerable impact on our stress level over the long term. Do you, or does your child, always have some kind of bug? Does even the smallest of health issues make you feel as if you're constantly doing battle with your own body? The study at Ohio State University is only one study, but it should encourage you to ask yourself some pointed questions about the kinds of inputs (stressors) you allow into your life on a regular basis.

I don't believe that television shows, movies, or videos alone can make you sick because there are too many contributing factors involved in maintaining a body's overall good health. But the question remains that we don't really know how much of a negative impact these types of things have. Because I personally notice that I react negatively when I watch a disturbing show on TV, I consciously choose to avoid those kinds of images whenever possible. I look for comedies or lighthearted movies instead. Even if I have seen a movie before (or a hundred times before, as my wife Kylee sometimes reminds me), if I know it's funny I'm willing to watch it again. I'm always up for a good laugh.

I typically only watch the news to see the weather forecast. Sure, I try to stay informed, but since most of the news these days reports on fires, murders, stabbings, shootings, kidnappings, rapes, car wrecks, and other sad and horrifying situations, why would I watch a lot of it? Why would anyone for that matter? It's my bet that if more people stop tuning in, we'd soon see the television stations and networks changing their tune and thinking about putting more positive stories on the air.

Do more and more people seem to be sick these days? I believe they are and that there are a number of reasons why. But I also believe that to be healthier individuals must begin to understand what is causing them to be in a state of "dis-ease," and make every effort possible to change the way they feel.

Keeping it simple

I think one of society's biggest problems is that we have forgotten how to keep things simple. We live at such a fast pace that it seems if we tried to slow down it would only make things worse. But slowing down might be the key to put things in much-needed perspective. A slower pace allows us to take the time we need, that our physical body, mind, and spirit need, to recognize what is going on inside us and around us. Looking within allows us to observe life more clearly, a state of mind that can help us begin to explore a more calm and peaceful existence.

How we approach life colors everything we feel, see, and do. It colors our relationships with other human beings and how we live each day. When our lives are frantic, when we don't take the time to "smell the roses," we can fall into patterns that keep us from experiencing life in a positive way. For example, a plant is an organic life form. Plants have specific colors, textures, size, fragrance, leaf patterns, and flowers, depending on the type. It is only when we apply our own individual subjectivity to plants that we imbue them with other characteristics. Our impressions, thoughts, preferences, and attitudes towards a plant are what makes it what it is for each of us. For example, a rose to one person may be beautiful and smell divinely sweet; to another it may be a thorny, allergy-inducing inconvenience. It is the same with art, where one person might look at a painting and love it, while another will think it's not worth the canvas it's painted on. The artwork itself isn't trying to be beautiful or unappealing; it simply is what it is—according to the eye of the beholder, who bases his or her judgment on a fully subjective opinion. And while opinions are important, they are neither inherently wrong or right; they do not make the painting or rose any more or less than it is on its own, regardless what anyone thinks.

It is my belief that we should try to be more like the rose or the painting—that is, to just BE in our natural state, with less effort and a more relaxed outlook.

One of my favorite quotes on the topic of effort is by the founder of the Functional Integration System of Neuromotor Education and Reconditioning, Mashe Feldenkrais, Ph.D. Dr. Feldenkrais said, "The sensation of effort is the subjective (personal) feeling of wasted movement. When an action is poorly and inefficiently performed, there is always a (personal) feeling of strain, friction or resistance. In an effort to perform an action more efficiently, one must generally *do less* and actually learn how not to make an effort." If we could learn how "not to make an effort," I think we would find we can also learn to live with less stress, and less stress can mean improved health all the way around.

29

How Stress & Cortisol "Steal" Your Hormones

We've been talking about stress and its relationship to the hormone cortisol. We said that when our bodies react to stress we produce more cortisol and that too much cortisol production can have numerous negative ramifications on the body over the long term. Cortisol production also has some positive effects, however, including the way it releases amino acids from muscle, glucose (sugar) from the liver, and fatty acids from fat into the bloodstream, all ways the body gets its energy. Cortisol production is what gets you bouncing out of bed and raring to go in the morning and what keeps you going throughout the day. As your cortisol level decreases, so does your energy, until you're ready for sleep at night. A low level of cortisol in the evening is appropriate because in that state your mind and body is preparing to relax so you can get a good night's sleep.

Circadian rhythm

The regular fluctuations in cortisol levels that we experience are referred to as the daily *circadian*, or *diurnal*, *rhythm*.

Typically, in any 24-hour period, the highest cortisol levels can be observed in the early morning and the lowest cortisol levels occur around midnight to 2:00 A.M.

*Circadian Rhythm.**

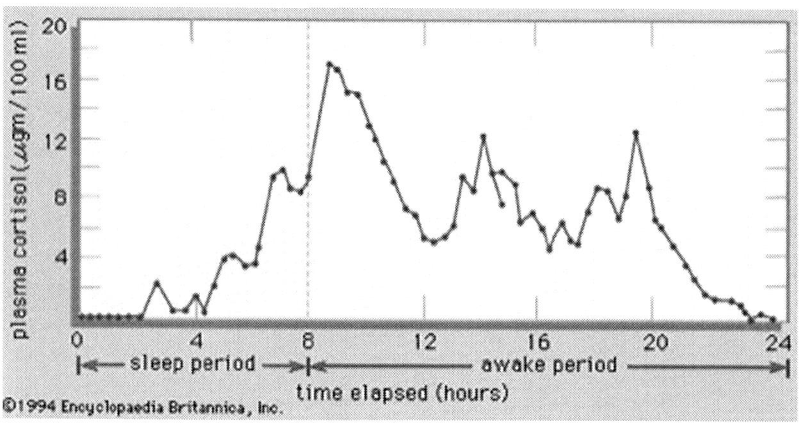

It is my experience that most people do not fit this natural pattern. In fact, they often have too much energy at the time they need it the least—when they retire at bedtime. If you ask them how they feel when they wake up, instead of saying they feel refreshed and looking forward to their day, they say they feel tired and worn out—even though they've just gotten out of bed. While there can be many reasons for this situation, a turn-around in the diurnal rhythm can be a primary indicator that their cortisol levels are higher than they should be—in other words, they are outside a proper rhythm and balance.

*Source: E. D. Weitzman, et al. 1971.*Twenty-four-hour Patterns of the Episodic Secretion of Cortisol in Normal Subjects*, *Journal of Clinical Endocrinology and Metabolism*, 33:13-22. Used with permission from The Endocrine Society, copyright 1971.

This is true for a number of patients we have tested in the clinic whose levels start out mid-range when they get up and return to about the same levels when they're ready to sleep. This means they are not getting that "boost" of cortisol when they need it in the morning and that they have too much at night when it's time to sleep. These patients have gone from "0 to 60" sometime long ago and their baseline now is in the 30 or 40 range, instead of at 0, where it needs to be. They are probably victims of what is referred to as the "cortisol steal," a topic I'll talk about shortly.

Cycles of imbalance

Unfortunately, many people attempt to offset the imbalance they feel with coffee, an energy drink, or some other stimulant to give them that kick-start they feel they need first thing in the morning. While it's true that these methods may work temporarily, the "crash" that comes mid-morning is an obvious downside. Crashing happens for two reasons: one, because the sugar that is usually included in these drinks makes insulin levels spike and then plummet, leaving you worse off than before and two, because the caffeine that entered your body gets processed and its effect is minimized as it leaves your system.

This mid-morning crash can also occur as a result of the type of breakfast you eat (or don't eat). Many of us start our day with processed carbohydrates like cereals, doughnuts or other sweet pastries, croissants, or bagels. Even if these carbs are wrapped around some type of protein (like that daily breakfast burrito or something-on-a-biscuit), the product is more than likely high in fat and full of chemicals. Hence, the reliable, annoyingly punctual, mid-morning crash. Of course, depending on what you eat for lunch, you'll experience the exact same scenario come mid-afternoon.

The best way to start your day is with some type of healthy protein, a small amount of fat, and a "good" carbohydrate source. The same advice applies to lunch. When you make these changes, you will notice a difference in your energy level and how you feel throughout the morning and throughout the day, probably from the very first day you start.

Nutrition and cortisol levels

Health care providers have known the benefits of a good breakfast for years. I'm sure you have heard more than once that breakfast is the most important meal of the day, and studies continue to be done that support this theory. One study, published in the journal *Pediatrics* ten years ago, for example, showed that kids who started off the day with a "bad carb" breakfast compared to one better balanced with protein and good carbs ate 81% more calories throughout the rest of the day. Although more recent studies have shown this number to be a bit lower, probably in the mid-60% range, either way that's a lot more calories—additional calories that lead to increased fat gain, especially if substantial exercise isn't used to offset the caloric intake. This is just another example of how nutrition plays a major role in helping to maintain proper hormone and cortisol levels.

Guyton's *Textbook of Medical Physiology*, used in medical schools across the country, states, "In the presence of great excesses of cortisol, the muscles can become so weak that the person cannot rise from the squatting position. And the immunity functions of the lymphoid tissue can be decreased to a small fraction of normal." Reading Guyton's statement makes me think of all of the patients, especially women, who present in my clinic with chronic fatigue, fibromyalgia, muscle weakness, and suppressed immune systems, and who tell me they have been looking everywhere for answers as to why they feel so crummy. I think of my own mom, who battled these conditions and symptoms for years and had test after test, none of which ever found the answer to why she felt the way she did.

Is it possible that the underlying cause of so many diverse symptoms is stress and the negative results stress wreaks on a body? I doubt that most of us are tested for stress when we go see our health care providers. But I believe it is not only possible, but probable, that stress is a major suspect for what ails us. The real challenge I see is that as an individual you can absolutely and positively affect your stress levels by how you think, feel, and act, as we have discussed. But if your hormone levels have been out of whack for potentially a very long time, positive change often requires getting the appropriate help from someone who can address your body's overall physical needs.

The "cortisol steal" and cholesterol

I referred to the "cortisol steal" a little earlier. In order to explain what this means, we first need to review how cortisol relates to cholesterol.

We've talked about how cholesterol—fat—gets a bad rap, but is vital to our survival and how "good" cholesterol is referred to as HDL (I think of the "H" as standing for "helper") and the "bad" cholesterol is called LDL ("L" because you want it to be low). We also know that because all hormones are made from cholesterol, we can safely assume that whether we call it cholesterol or fat it serves a positive purpose—as long as we don't have too much.

But too little fat can be a problem as well. One example is girls who are athletes, like long-distance runners, who have very little body fat. It has been shown that a significantly low percentage of body fat can interfere with normal hormone production and that girls who undertake a high level of regular physical activity often experience a delay in their menstrual periods or have irregular cycles.

Since during extended periods of heightened stress cortisol levels remain constantly elevated, the cortisol produced needs access to more and more cholesterol. In order to get it, it basically "steals" it from the other hormones. The result is that more cortisol and less of all the other hormones, like progesterone, estrogen, DHEA, and testosterone, is produced.

Think of the cortisol steal as a faucet with two hoses attached. The faucet is the cortisol and the two attached hoses connect to other hormones in the body (like estrogen, progesterone, DHEA, and testosterone). When the cortisol steal is underway, it's as if someone is tightening the faucet, gradually slowing the flow to the hoses leading to the other hormones. If the conditions in the body that started the steal go on long enough, the cortisol faucet will begin to shut itself off. If this continues, only a trickle will be getting through to the other hormones. At that point, the majority of the body's cholesterol will be going only to the faucet; that is, only to the cortisol (see the next page for a diagram of the "cortisol steal in action").

In effect, the cortisol is taking what it needs to stay elevated to deal with your stress, but leaving your body without the other hormones it needs to feel good, function properly, and stay healthy. You are virtually being held hostage from inside your own body. This is yet another reason why it is vitally important for you to do all you can to control your stress and to get help when you need it for the things you can't do yourself.

The "cortisol steal."

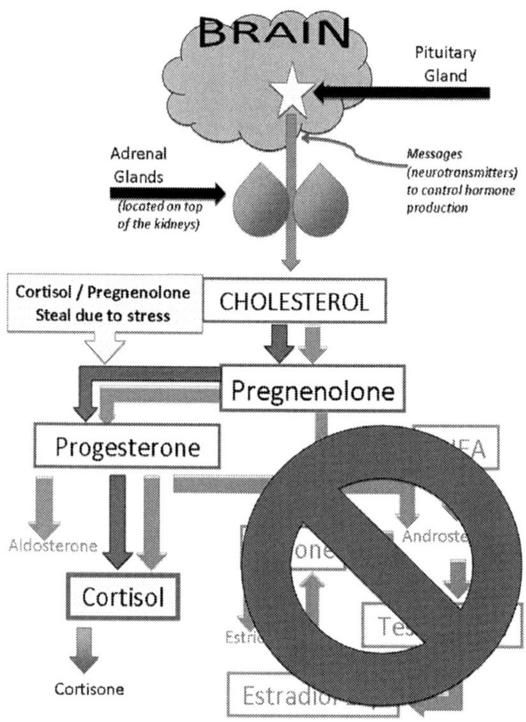

Getting help with stress obviously includes dealing with your cortisol levels, but it's equally as important to address your other hormone levels as well. Sometimes more than one type of health care professional is needed to rectify symptoms from a hormonal imbalance like this. Professionals may include primary care physicians, endocrinologists, gynecologists, chiropractors, psychologists, psychiatrists, acupuncturists, and others.

The most important thing to remember is to never take "I don't know," "It's all in your head," or "You'll just have to live with it"—or any other response that makes you feel like there is no hope—for an answer. No matter how significant or insignificant your conditions or symptoms may appear to others, they are yours. You are the one who has been living with them and only you know how you feel. Only you know how they have been affecting your ability to live life to the fullest. Most of us would agree that just getting by is not good enough and that if the same old approach with the same lack of results doesn't work it's time to try something new and to try that something new as soon as possible.

30

"DAD, REMEMBER THE TIME I ALMOST KILLED YOU?"

Remember my story about how I suffered the consequences of waiting too long to find the reason for my collapse? Do you recall how I promised myself that I would learn to "control my stress"? You probably assumed that I'd learned my lesson and that I lived happily ever after, right?

Wrong.

Not so fast. After all, I had spent a long time ignoring all the problems that got me where I was; how could I expect them to go away overnight and without a fight?

Here is what really happened. Shortly after my wife Kylee and I met we took Alex down to the pool in the apartment complex where I was living at the time. I had filled Kylee in on the generalities of what had happened regarding what I now thought of as "my heart episode," but I hadn't told her any of the specifics. Why? I told myself it was because they weren't pertinent. After all, that period of my life was behind me. Right?

Wrong again.

Alex and I were enjoying some relief from the hot summer sun in the pool while Kylee soaked up a few rays on one the chairs pool side. Alex was 6 or so at the time and full of energy. "Let's see who can swim the longest under the water, Dad," she said, excited to compete against me in an event we both knew she would win. She knew she'd win because she could swim a long way under water, probably farther than anyone in the whole world. I knew she'd win because I was her dad. And so, on the count of three, we would hold our breath and swim as far as we could. I counted, "One, twoooo, THREE," and Alex promptly filled her little lungs with air and began her swim to victory. I, too, filled my lungs with air, simultaneously going under the water. And that's when I felt it, the all too familiar thump in my chest. Suddenly my heart was hammering its arhythmic beat to an uncharted course. I immediately surfaced to see Alex wiping the water from her eyes a short distance away. Her face was lit with pride and victory for a moment. Then the light switched off as she detected something wasn't right. I made my way as calmly as I could to the edge of the pool and gently eased myself out.

I approached Kylee and informed her of what I thought. Correction, what I knew. Out loud I said I hoped I was wrong, but we immediately went back to my apartment, where I confirmed my diagnosis with my stethoscope. Kylee was terrified.

It had been selfish, foolish, and irresponsible not to fully explain what I had experienced in Austin, given the fact that I knew it could happen again. Sharing the information would have saved time and hard feelings and, most importantly, Kylee would have known what to do. But I hadn't said anything and I could see she was panicking, albeit silently, probably the way I had months before.

We quickly went to the car and Kylee got behind the wheel. She was now still quiet, but clearly bordering on hysterical, so much so that I had to give her directions to a hospital she knew well and that was less than two miles away. Kylee shared with me later that it wasn't that she didn't know how to get to the hospital, but that in her mind she was running through what she would do when I lost consciousness and my heart stopped beating. How would she keep me alive, drive to the hospital, deal with Alex, and address her own fears all at the same time? (It took me a while to forgive myself for having been so selfish. I knew the routine, while she had no idea what might be in store. I was being such a *guy*. I admit to marrying way over my head. Sorry, Kylee, and thank you.)

Fortunately for all of us, I remained conscious all the way to the hospital, but it took the entire afternoon and evening in the emergency room before I was admitted. Of course, my heart was still in a-fib so they couldn't release me. Same routine: IV drugs to help reset my heart to its normal rhythm or I would be subjected to the dreaded shock cart, the one I had so narrowly managed to avoid in Austin. The doctor who was caring for me put it in a different way. "If your heart doesn't revert to natural rhythm on its own, we will apply a gentle current across your chest to help it."

What? Current is electricity and we are all taught at a very young age you don't play with electricity. Gentle, schmentle. Was this guy crazy? I knew exactly what he meant and let him know it, but thanked him for explaining it so pleasantly. It was as if my heart knew what was in store for if it didn't cooperate, because then, right on cue, it did what it had done in Austin and reverted to normal early in the morning before the "gentle current" was to be applied.

This episode was definitely on the mild side compared to the last one because my body didn't suffer the severity of side effects that occur when the heart doesn't work as it should for a much longer period of time. I'd come through this one in pretty good shape. Kylee, on the other hand, and Alex, as I would later learn, had not.

Given Kylee's love and concern for me, she was tormented by thoughts of all that could go wrong in the future—in essence, she was focusing on all the worst-case scenarios and what they would mean to her life with me. We worked hard to communicate until we both felt more at ease with the circumstances and to this day she is unbelievably supportive.

Without a doubt, though, the most difficult realization for me came when I learned how traumatized Alex had been at the time.

It was several years later when she and I were riding in the car. I don't remember the conversation that led up to her comment, probably because I was so shocked, horrified, and saddened by what she asked.

"Dad, do you remember when I almost killed you?"

I don't take particular pleasure in admitting this, but it's altogether true and Kylee will confirm it. I don't feel as badly about anything, and I mean anything, as when I feel I have let Alex down or when she is upset for any reason. The connection we have is so strong that often my moods mirror hers or vice versa. If she's feeling good, so do I; if she's not, I can feel my own mental state take a dive. I have had to work very hard over the years to manage the level of *simpatico*, or empathy, I share with Alex, because I know there is no value in not being able to manage it. But it has been tough. And to hear that my little girl thought she was responsible for what happened to me—even more, that she believed she had almost killed me...well, it ripped my heart out.

Fighting back tears, I asked, "What did you say?" I needed to buy a little time to gain some clarity, to verify that what I heard was what Alex had actually said. Unfortunately, it was. Alex said again, "Remember the time in the pool when I almost killed you?" The second time wasn't any easier or clearer. It hit me just as hard as the first.

"Oh, no. No, no, Alex. It wasn't your fault, you didn't cause what happened." I said this with as much conviction as I'd ever said anything before in my life. I proceeded to lay out, in as basic terms as I could, what had happened to my heart and why I'd had to be in the hospital. I pleaded with her to understand that the things that had happened to me were in my control and no one else's. That neither she nor anyone else could make me have heart problems—at least not of the physical kind. I hoped she was listening.

I continued to remind Alex over the next several months that she hadn't caused what had happened in the pool that day, that she was just there when it happened. You never know if kids tell you what they believe or what they want you to believe. I keep hoping, though, that she told me the truth when she acknowledged she understood that she had nothing to do with it.

…

I started on a long journey to de-stress my life. In hindsight, I can easily see that all the little clues I'd gotten through the years, all the indicators that something bad was about to happen, had slipped by me because I had let them. It was convenient to assume none of these hints were connected because that meant I could ignore them completely.

Once I changed my outlook, I knew I needed to see everything in a different light. Now I spend a great deal of time reading and listening to CDs on a variety of topics, including positive thinking, mediation, spirituality, and anything else I think will help keep me headed in the right direction. I have spent more time in the last ten years than I spent in the 30 years before that figuring out who I really am and answering a lot of life's questions as they pertain to me. That effort, along with some significant lifestyle changes, has changed my life, where I can honestly say I have never been happier, less stressed, more at ease, and more connected with who and what I am, as well as with the people around me.

So whatever it takes for you, maybe it's a little event or a big sign, don't ignore it the way I did and so many others do until something REALLY big happens. Don't wait for your door to be kicked in when the circus comes to town. Pay attention and respond to what your body and mind are telling you, because that gut feeling you get might just save your life.

CONCLUSION

LIVING THE LIFE YOU WERE GIFTED TO LIVE

As I said in the very beginning of *Hormone Basics*, whether you are 14, 44, or 114, you are neither too young nor too old to learn what you need to know to change your life. I trust that with what you now know about hormones and your understanding of how you and your body fit into the bigger picture of living a healthy life, you will have lots to do. If there are still some areas that have you a bit confused, don't be concerned—you always have the option to pursue more clarity as you learn more and more about your body. One of the great advantages of the human body is that the basic fundamentals of its mechanisms never really change that much—and this includes hormones. If and when you do find yourself looking for more information and resources, please start at our website, www.hormonebasics.com.

Here is an overview of what I hope you will take away from reading this book.

The human body is a complex system of organs, arteries, veins, bones, muscles, nerves, chemicals, hormones, and more. In an ideal world, this system has the ability to function perfectly so that we experience perfect emotional, mental, and physical health.

In reality, because this is not an ideal world, this complex system often suffers setbacks or malfunctions. Sometimes these setbacks occur early on, originating from the birthing process itself, or later as we inevitably experience what life throws at us in the form of accidents, toxins, nutritional deficits, stress, and so on. Ultimately, if the setbacks we experience continue unchecked, they can take a devastating toll on every aspect of our health.

One of the most significant aspects of the way the human body works is hormones, as they play a huge role in the overall health and functioning of this vast system.

Because hormones are the heart and driving force of the amazing and wonderful system you know as "you," one could easily say that in essence, you *are* your hormones. These microscopic chemical messengers that control every one of the gazillions of things going on inside you every second are at the center of everything that happens in the body on all levels. Your hormones control how good you feel, how healthy you are, how clearly you think, how much energy you have, how much you accomplish, how long you live, the quality of life you have…we could go on and on. Suffice it to say that hormones affect every single amazing, incredible, indescribable attribute that makes you the unique individual you are and were meant to be.

That's why, if you feel you are being controlled by your hormones in a way that has cast you into a state of dis-ease—something you should now be able to ascertain from the lists of symptoms of hormone imbalance in this book—don't ignore that feeling! The key is to understand your hormonal makeup in the context of your body and then to find a health care provider who is willing to explore any findings with you.

Once we develop a deep understanding of the myriad ways that hormones affect us, we can make larger decisions about how to live our lives more healthfully and productively so as to achieve the highest possible quality of life. We can start by shifting our thinking from that of a victim to that of an advocate of environmental safety and health safety for everyone on the planet. When we do find an imbalance in our bodies, we can make efforts to correct it. When we feel angry about the way we've been treated in the past or frustrated by the toxic environment we have created, we can put that energy towards creating a better place. The real test is whether or not we will choose to make different decisions based on the information we have. The journey to better health starts with us, because we can't take care of others effectively until we care for ourselves. And frankly, we are never too busy to care for ourselves if we make that a top priority.

Convincing ourselves we are "too busy" to take care of ourselves only allows us to go on doing the same things and getting the same results. So, even though food is as close as the next supermarket, drive-through, or microwave, and…

…even though the chemicals used to make our clothes, our furniture, our houses, and our medicines are known to be toxic and…

…even though these products, foods, and drugs can cause more negative side-effects than positive corrections to our health and wellbeing and…

…even though we are being robbed of our good health one step at a time…

We have the choice to change the way we live.

…

Finally, there are two things that will remain constant throughout your life as a woman: you are female and you have hormones. But it is in your control to affect changes within the context of those physical parameters. When you know that something is "off," you can choose to continue to ignore it or choose to be ignored by those around you. It is my belief that you are too important and too loved for this to be the case. If you don't feel that way, it may be because your mind, body, and spirit have not received what they need to blossom.

I also believe there are two basic ways to view life: as a life you are living or a life that is dying. You are either alive and living life to its fullest or you are not, and if you are not living life to the fullest you have chosen the dying option. Of course not dying isn't really an option seeing as we all die eventually. But the way we live is a choice we make every day.

I will end this book the way I began, by saying that THERE IS HOPE! Never stop believing in this truth and never stop searching for your own personal answers, because no one else can do it for you. Because your path to finding the answers you want will not be exactly the same as that of your classmate, coworker, family member, friend, or neighbor, be prepared to follow your own path on this journey and let your heart guide you. Know that you are never alone, that there is always someone waiting to help you. Love yourself enough to want to feel better and be healthier and know there are plenty of us out here who care about you and want the same for you.

I've written this book to help you find your way to better health and to truly enjoy the great life you were gifted to live. Enjoying life can start right now—today—when you start taking the time to continue to educate yourself about the workings of your mind, body, and spirit, and empowering yourself by applying what you've learned. It all makes a difference. My advice? Eat, drink, and live as healthily as you can as much of the time as you can. Detoxify your mind and your body on a consistent and continual basis and find those of us in the health care profession who will join you in caring for you and your health. If you want to find out more about what you have read in this book, visit my website, www.hormonebasics.com. I've loaded it with information that can help you feel good, both inside and out.

What are my hopes for you?

That you will start by having one good day—*one day*—of feeling good. Then two…and then three.

That your days will go from good to great. When that happens, I know with certainty that you will start to feel more competent and more able to focus on YOU and on the things that are important to you. Things like family, career, and school…in other words, all the things that matter when you don't spend all your time thinking about what's "wrong with you."

That you will be able to follow your gift, to live from your soul, and grow through your heart.

That you will become more dedicated to and empowered by your health and that you will learn to control your life and your health—not have them control you.

And finally, above all else, it is my hope that when you start living the life you were gifted to live, you will love the life you are living—forever.

About the Author

Raised in Ponca City, Oklahoma and educated at Oklahoma State University and Cleveland Chiropractic College, Chris Leatherman, D.C., FASA studied under the tutelage of Dr. Richard Yennie, recipient of the World Health Organization's Man of the Year award. Dr. Leatherman is board-certified by the National Board of Chiropractic Examiners and the states of Missouri and Kansas; is a member of the Acupuncture Society of America, the International Chiropractic Pediatric Association (ICPA), and the New Medicine Foundation; is a certified First Line Therapy (FLT) therapeutic lifestyle health care provider, and past president of the board of directors for The Body Composition Clinics, Inc. Professional affiliations include the Pinnacle Management Group. He is also certified in the Webster Technique, a chiropractic technique for pregnant mothers developed by Dr. Larry Webster, founder of ICPA.

Dr. Leatherman spends his time seeing patients in his busy Kansas City, Missouri and Overland Park, Kansas chiropractic clinics and educating on the topics of chiropractic care, hormones, and natural health at seminars from Atlanta to San Diego. An avid advocate for women's health, Dr. Leatherman has made it his prime objective to help as many people as he can live the lives they were gifted to live. Dr. Leatherman is happily married to his wife Kylee and proud dad to his daughter Alex and son Bobby.

Dr. Leatherman can be reached at:
THE LEATHERMAN CLINIC
Gentle Chiropractic
Phone: 816.637.5000
Email: info@hormonebasics.com
Clinic Website: www.4tlc.com

To purchase copies of **Hormone Basics,**
please go to www.hormonebasics.com.